The Modern Rise
of Population

The Modern Rise of Population

Thomas McKeown

Edward Arnold

© Thomas McKeown 1976

First published 1976 by
Edward Arnold (Publishers) Ltd
25 Hill Street, London W1X 8LL

ISBN 0 7131 5867 0

Printed in Great Britain by
Butler & Tanner Ltd, Frome and London

Contents

1
The problem and the approach

Since this book is concerned with the modern rise of population it will be desirable at the outset to clarify the sense in which this term is used. It will be taken to refer to the growth of population which began in the late seventeenth or early eighteenth century and has continued to the present day. And while the discussion will be based on European, and particularly British, experience, it is the remarkable increase in world population as a whole that it seeks to explain.

Although all estimates of world population are subject to a considerable error, the basic facts are not in doubt. During most of his time on earth, man has lived as a nomad, dependent for his food on hunting, fishing and gathering of fruit. Under such conditions the earth supported no more than a few people per square mile, and it has been estimated that when cultivation and domestication of plants and animals began about 10,000 years ago, the total population was below, and probably well below, 10 million. By 1750 when the modern rise had just began, the number had increased to 750 million; it was 1000 million in 1830, 2000 in 1930, 3000 in 1960 and 4000 in 1975 (figure 1.1). That is to say, it took hundreds of thousands of years for the human population to expand to the first thousand million; the second was added in 100 years, the third in 30 and the fourth in 15.

The growth of population in England and Wales was even more remarkable. It is shown in figure 1.2, from the eleventh century when it was estimated as one and a half million by a count of families for the Domesday Book. The population increased to five and a half million in 1700, 18 in 1851 and 49 in 1971. For investigation of population growth, English data have two important advantages: one, that the modern increase appears to have begun somewhat earlier than in other countries; the other, that cause of death, which is critical for population study, was recorded nationally on death certificates from 1838. Elsewhere this information was not available before the late nineteenth century.

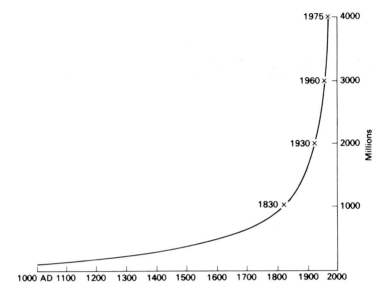

1.1 The modern rise of world population.

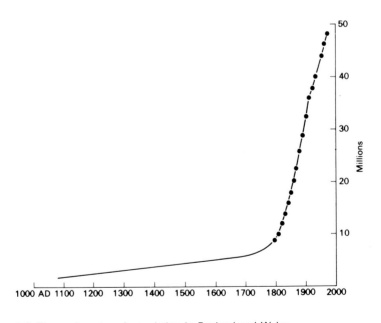

1.2 The modern rise of population in England and Wales.

Although the modern rise of population has received, and continues to receive, a great deal of attention, the main interest has been in its implications for the future. Estimates based on recent trends have given alarming figures for the size of populations to be expected in the year 2000 and beyond, and it is understandable that discussion has been focused on the reliability of the estimates, their implications with regard to the limits of food and other resources, and the steps which might be taken to reduce the rate of growth. However, the reasons for the increase of population have had relatively little attention, and it has been assumed rather than demonstrated that it was associated broadly with advances in medicine and improved living conditions. There has been no serious attempt to establish the time when these influences became effective, or to distinguish between the very different effects of increased food supplies, improvements in hygiene and the prevention and treatment of disease in the individual. Interpretation is particularly confused by the practice of grouping together hygiene, immunization and therapy under the term 'medical measures'. For although doctors have contributed to all three, it is important to separate changes in the physical environment from specific preventive and therapeutic measures applied to the individual. In concluding that the modern rise of population has not so far been considered in sufficient depth, I do not of course overlook the large literature in historical demography; however this is concerned mainly with the initial phase of population growth, particularly in the eighteenth century, rather than with the increase from the late seventeenth century to the present day as a whole.

It is not difficult to suggest reasons for this omission. Medical historians have largely ignored the modern growth of population and economic historians have dealt with only a part of it. From the point of view of the economic historian the crucial issue in demography is the relation between population growth and industrial and economic development. He asks, 'Did the Industrial Revolution create its own labour force?' – a pithy way of enquiring whether improved economic conditions led to an expansion of population, or whether the growth of population which assisted industrialization was due to some other cause essentially independent of it. This interest has led historians to focus attention on the pre-registration period and they have been less concerned with the demography after 1838, when the explanation of population growth has seemed more obvious. Still less have they attempted to explain the modern increase of population as a whole, an omission which arises also from the fact that most of those interested in the problem and period tend to work on either the eighteenth or the nineteenth century. It is not history but historians who are divisible by centuries.

The approach of medical historians to the subject has been quite different. They have investigated the behaviour of individual diseases, particularly infectious diseases, and a good deal has been written about the decline of mortality from tuberculosis, smallpox, typhus, scarlet fever and some other infections. But the medical historian has had little incentive to consider the decline of mortality as a whole, and while by remaining silent he may seem to have endorsed explanations suggested by economic historians, he has really ignored them. The interpretation of the contribution of medical influences to the reduction of mortality and improvement in health has not been a theme of medical history in the way that eighteenth-century population growth has been a theme of economic history.

At this point it should be said that an understanding of the modern rise of population is linked closely to an understanding of the modern transformation in man's health. Although they cannot be shown to be exactly coincident, both changes have occurred in – to give an outside limit – the past three centuries. Investigation of population growth leads inescapably to consideration of the trend of mortality and of the behaviour of individual diseases (mainly the infections); and interpretation of the improvement in health makes it essential to consider the reasons for the increase of population in the period before births, deaths and cause of death were registered nationally.

The rise of population and the associated transformation of health are among the great themes of history, in interest and importance perhaps second only to the origin of life. The effects on human life, most for good but some also for ill, have already been profound. The future consequences, if population growth is not soon restricted, may be disastrous. For practical purposes, therefore, as well as intrinsic interest, it is essential to seek an explanation of the increase of population. Ideally such an explanation should not only indentify the more important influences which have been at work; it should also assess their contributions to the growth of population and improvement in health and, so far as possible, suggest the time from which they have been effective.

This enquiry is not one for the faint-hearted. There are no data which put the issues wholly beyond dispute, nor – to express a personal opinion – are they likely ever to become available. It is true that many countries are awaiting the industrial and sanitary revolutions with accompanying improvement in standard of living, literacy and health as well as increase of population, and at first sight it might seem possible to interpret this experience in the light of present-day knowledge, using modern statistical and other evidence. But we shall not see a repetition of the circumstances which existed in the western world between the end of the seventeenth century and the beginning of the twentieth, for it is already clear that the order and, perhaps, the magnitude of the main influences – nutritional, hygienic and therapeutic – will not be the same. The choice in respect of the historical question is not therefore between a correct and an incorrect answer; it is between the best answer that can be given and none at all. This being so, many people, and particularly biologists who are used to working with more reliable data, will prefer to leave the research to others with a greater tolerance of uncertainty. It would be unfortunate if this led to the continued neglect of one of the major themes of history.

THE APPROACH

Since the problem is complex and the data are deficient, it is essential at the outset to decide how it should be tackled. I think there is no doubt that in the past the approach has been inadequate in at least two respects. In the first place, attention has been focused on only part of the problem, the rise of population in the eighteenth and early nineteenth centuries. And secondly, this subject has often been investigated without sufficient regard for later, and in general more reliable, evidence and experience. The failure to take account of present-day knowledge has been particularly serious in appraisal of the contribution of medical measures and of the behaviour of infections diseases. For example, we are unlikely to make a reliable judgement about reasons for the decline of smallpox in the eighteenth century if we are unaware of the means of its control in the twentieth.

I suggest that a more satisfactory basis for study is as follows. First, the subject for investigation should be the modern increase of population as a whole rather than its initial phase. Second, we should examine the evidence from the time when births, deaths and cause of death were recorded nationally before turning to the uncertainties of the pre-registration period. And third the approach should be comprehensive rather than fragmented; as an illustration, in order to determine the time from which medical intervention contributed significantly to the control of disease, we should consider all the information, present as well as past, rather than rely on interpretation of the trend of single diseases, particularly in the eighteenth century. These suggestions are developed in the discussion which follows.

The modern rise of population considered as a whole

Throughout man's history, population size has fluctuated, at times widely, mainly in response to variation in mortality. While direct observations are lacking, it seems probable that numbers increased substantially whenever the conditions of life improved, for example after cultivation and domestication of plants and animals at the time of the first agricultural revolution and again, for less obvious reasons, in Britain in the twelfth, thirteenth and sixteenth centuries.

It is important to decide whether the modern rise is to be regarded as analogous to these earlier increases, given particular but not necessarily unique significance because of its coincidence with the Industrial Revolution. If so, it seems permissible to argue by analogy and to invoke the same kinds of explanations as are proposed for earlier periods. This treatment has been adopted by some historians when they attribute the eighteenth-century increase to a decline of mortality, brought about by cyclic changes in the behaviour of infectious diseases or even of a single disease such as plague. But if the modern increase was essentially different from earlier population changes so too, we should expect, must be the reasons for it.

The modern rise of population is distinguished clearly from all previous increases by three things – its size, its continuity and its duration. The scale of the changes shown in figures 1.1 and 1.2 leaves no doubt that we are dealing with a unique phenomenon; but also, unlike any previous rise, it has continued without interruption for nearly three centuries, and a major challenge of our times is to bring it to an end.

Since the modern rise is unique, it is quite unsatisfactory to attempt to explain separately its initial phase. In Britain it probably began in the eighteenth century; it was well advanced before births and deaths were registered, and even by the time of the first census in 1801, the increase in numbers was much greater than that which occurred in earlier periods. For the purpose of interpreting the modern increase of population it is unnecessary, and probably impossible, to state precisely when it started. It is sufficient to know that whatever the trend in the early years of the eighteenth century, at some time well before its end the unique expansion had begun.

Reasons for beginning with the post-registration period
If the basic data were available it would seem natural to begin the study of the modern rise of population with its onset in the eighteenth century. Unfortunately the data are not available, and it is hardly possible to read the literature of the past two decades without being acutely aware of the deficiencies. Estimates before and after the eighteenth century leave no doubt that the population of England and Wales increased substantially during that period, but this is perhaps the only point about which there is general agreement. It is not known when the increase began; the relative contributions of a rise in the birth rate and a fall in the death rate are still disputed; and although ingenious hypotheses have been constructed on assumptions about the behaviour of single diseases, the causes of mortality remain unknown.

The deficiencies of evidence have not gone unrecognized. Flinn was

particularly explicit: 'The only *facts* of national population growth
are still the figures derived from nineteenth-century censuses and the
civil registration of births, marriages and deaths after 1838' and, 'the
really important advance in the scholarship of recent years is that for
the first time in the study of Britain's population in the eighteenth
century we recognize that we know so little.'[1] This recognition has not
deterred investigators from pursuing their enquiries in the pre-
registration period, and where the field of discussion has been extended,
it has often been back to earlier centuries for which the evidence is
even less secure.

For investigation of population growth we need to know not only
population size, but also the birth rate, death rate and cause of death.
The birth rate and death rate are required in order to assess the
contribution of an increase of the one or a decrease of the other to
population growth – the issue which has had so much attention in
eighteenth-century studies; and cause of death is essential for appraisal
of reasons for the decline of mortality. In England and Wales these
minimal data are available nationally only after 1838.

Demographers and historians interested in the pre-registration
period have attempted to provide a substitute for national records by
exploiting the information available on parish registers and bills of
mortality. Can we, from such sources, expect to get a reliable national
estimate of fertility, mortality and cause of death? I do not think so.

Parish registers record baptisms, marriages and burials and, while
in some places registers may be complete to the beginning of civil
registration in 1837, too few now exist to permit assembly of an accurate
national picture from them. At a national level, estimates of population
and population changes during the eighteenth century are based on
the returns obtained to a question in the 1801 census, asking for the
number of baptisms and burials in each 'Parish, Township or Place'
for each decadal year from 1700 to 1780 and for every year from then
until 1800. Thus, for the greater part of the eighteenth century there
are figures only for every tenth year, some of which are recognized
to be exceptional from a demographic point of view.

Even at the time of the census, however, the registers on which the
returns were based were known to be incomplete in the registration
of baptisms and burials, and to obtain national estimates allowance
has to be made for unregistered births and deaths. 'The estimates for
birth and death rates are highly sensitive to the allowances that the
particular estimator thinks fit to make, and the evidence on this point
is so scanty that we do not know within a very wide margin what

1 M. W. Flinn, *British Population Growth, 1700–1850*. Economic History Society (London, 1970),
p. 50.

the right allowance would be.'[2] Chambers noted that for the period prior to Lord Hardwicke's Marriage Act of 1753, 'it is impossible to make a valid statement about the rate of marriage from the study of a single parish' and, 'the difficulties in the way of calculating the rate of birth to which the marriages gave rise is even greater.'[3]

To complicate matters further, the accuracy of individual registers varied from year to year. After a critical review of parish sources, Krause concluded 'that parochial registration was relatively accurate in the early eighteenth century, became somewhat less so in the 1780s, virtually collapsed between roughly 1795 and 1820 and then improved somewhat between 1821 and 1837.'[4] However, even this appraisal must be viewed with caution: a report of 1774 on the population of Manchester states 'this account does not include the deaths, or births, amongst the Dissenters. These, by a late improvement in our bills of mortality, are now admitted into the parish register.'[5] How 'late' the improvement is we are not told, but on figures averaged over the previous five years, it has the effect of raising the number of deaths by nearly 6 per cent, and of births by over 18 per cent. Presumably at some earlier period Dissenters were not included, though how much earlier and whether they contributed proportionately in the same way to births and deaths is unknown.

It is indeed difficult to assess the reliability of the registers at any time during the eighteenth century. The allowances needed for under-registration must have varied from place to place and from year to year, and are still in dispute. But in any case, the undoubted variation in fertility and mortality from one area to another makes it most unlikely that an acceptable national picture could result from the study of individual registers.

The use of the bills of mortality to determine the reasons for the decline in mortality depends on the completeness, or failing that the representativeness, of their coverage, and on the value of a layman's assessment of cause of death in the eighteenth century. The London bills are the most widely known; but bills were also compiled for other places, both urban and rural, and a book was devoted to a discussion of them.[6] However, it is clear from this and other comments that they were not compiled for every town or parish, and that coverage of the

---

[2] H. J. Habakkuk, 'The economic history of modern Britain'. In *Population in History*, edited by D. V. Glass and D. E. C. Eversley, Arnold (London, 1965), p. 149.

[3] J. D. Chambers, *Population, Economy and Society in Pre-Industrial Britain*. Oxford University Press (London, 1972), p. 59.

[4] J. T. Krause, 'The changing adequacy of English registration, 1600–1837'. In *Population in History*, op. cit., p. 393.

[5] T. Percival, 'Observations on the state of population in Manchester'. *Philosophical Transactions of the Royal Society*, **64** (1774).

[6] T. Short, 'New observations on City, Town and Country Bills of Mortality, etc.' (1750).

whole country was quite incomplete.[7] Since this is so, it is unlikely that the bills which do exist can be used to represent the mortality experience of the whole country. In relation to total mortality at least, the experience was very different between towns for which bills were compiled. 'The slightest survey, of the following Tables, will manifestly show how erroneous and unjust every calculation, relating to this subject, must be, drawn from the London bills, or perhaps those of most other considerable towns, and applied to the inhabitants of this city. Chester is healthy to a most uncommon degree.'[8] If the overall mortality is so different, so too must be the distribution of the causes of death; the extent to which these differences are maintained when considering localities for which bills are not available is quite unknown, and to assemble a national picture from existing bills would be even more difficult than from parish registers.

The imperfections and inaccuracies in the diagnosed causes of death have been recognized since Graunt made the first observations in 1662. 'The knowledge even of the numbers which die of the Plague is not sufficiently deduced from the meer Reports of the Searchers... For we shall make it probable, that in the Years of Plague, a quarter part more dies of that disease than are set down.' However, he was not unduly concerned that the bills should be meticulously accurate. 'I say, it is enough, if we know from the Searchers but the most predominant Symptoms' and, 'in case a man of seventy-five years old died of a Cough ... I esteem it little error ... if this Person be ... reckoned among the Aged, and not placed under the Title of Cough.' He acknowledged that there were 'those Casualties, which are aptest to be confounded and mistaken', and considered that the searchers were 'perhaps, ignorant and careless'. More recent work has also shown that the searchers were not above taking a bribe to make a false return as to the cause of death, though whether this occurred on a scale large enough to have any influence on the overall distribution of causes of mortality is doubtful.

In the eighteenth century the system of recording cause of death in some places differed slightly from that used in London, and parish clerks rather than searchers made the enquiries. This does not seem to have resulted in much improvement in diagnosis. 'With respect to the general Table of Diseases, the obvious uncertainties and inaccuracy of an enquiry which, in most cases would only be made by the clerk in the churchyard, made me despair of rendering it in any great degree subservient to the purposes of science' and, 'the alarming article of

---

[7] J. Dodson, 'A letter concerning an improvement in the Bills of Mortality'. *Philosophical Transactions of the Royal Society*, **47** (1751-2).

[8] J. Haygarth, 'Observations on the Bill of Mortality at Chester for the year 1772'. *Philosophical Transactions of the Royal Society*, **64** (1774).

Consumption, which includes all those returned under the common terms of Weakness, Surfeit and Decay, has been arranged under three different periods of age, to enable the medical reader the better to judge of the different diseases contained under it.'[9]

Heberden, frankly incredulous that the numbers of deaths ascribed to measles could be so high, considered that 'the scarlet fever and malignant sore throat . . . may easily be mistaken for measles by better judges than the mothers and nurses', while Farr, in the first report of the Registrar General, seems finally to have refuted any claims to accuracy that the bills may have had when he wrote that 'each disease has in many instances been denoted by three or four terms, and each term has been applied to as many different diseases; vague, inconvenient names have been employed, or complications have been registered instead of primary diseases.'

In summary, a present-day assessment of the bills of mortality would be roughly as follows. One cannot even now be satisfied with certification of cause of death. Nineteenth-century post-registration data must be approached with considerable reservations, by asking separately about each disease whether we can rely on a clinical diagnosis unsupported by laboratory or other evidence. We can therefore have little confidence in discussions of the trend of individual diseases in the eighteenth century, when national records were not available and death was certified by a layman; and for earlier centuries assessment of the behaviour of diseases can be little more than guesswork.

Since the basic data are not available before 1838 in England and Wales, it seems essential to begin enquiry after that time, when there is sufficient information to support a hypothesis. Fortunately the problem of extrapolating from the later to the earlier period is in some respects less difficult than might be supposed. For example, if in the light of knowledge of the diseases which declined after 1838, it is concluded that immunization and therapy did not contribute to the reduction of the death rate before 1900, it seems reasonable to assume that such measures are very unlikely to have been effective a hundred years earlier. As it is known that a decline of bowel infections coincided with the introduction of sanitary measures in the nineteenth century, we can be fairly confident that improved hygiene was not a significant influence during the eighteenth. And if a reminder is needed that mortality from a single infection may fluctuate, apparently without medical or other intervention, in a period when other influences are changing the whole pattern of disease, it is provided by experience of scarlet fever in the nineteenth and twentieth centuries.

[9] J. Aikin, 'The Bill of Mortality for the town of Warrington'. *Philosophical Transactions of the Royal Society*, **64** (1774).

A comprehensive approach

If we accept that the modern rise of population should be considered as a whole and that it is desirable to begin with the later period when births, deaths and cause of death were registered, the question remains as to the best way to tackle it. A metaphor may make it easier to see the alternatives. Should we think of the problem as a jig-saw, in which individual pieces prepared by careful research are finally fitted together to form a complete and perhaps unexpected picture? Or should we regard it as a canvas on which a comprehensive inter-pretation is sketched at an early stage, later detailed work being used to fill in and modify the outline where this proves necessary? The first is the generally accepted approach but I think there are good reasons for preferring the second.

At first sight the jig-saw approach looks attractive, even essential. Given the grave limitations of the evidence, particularly in the early period, is it not necessary to exploit fully eighteenth-century sources which may throw light on fertility, mortality and causes of death, and in the meantime to keep our heads down and refuse to speculate too far until we can be more confident about the quality of the data? This approach is well illustrated by the two scholarly essays which introduced *Population in History*, an extensive collection of papers concerned mainly with the demography of the eighteenth and early nineteenth centuries.[10] The programme of research outlined there is formidable indeed, comprising a vast range of multinational projects of almost unlimited scope and duration. Viewed in this way, the demo-graphy of the past three centuries is hardly a subject on which we can expect early answers to the main questions; it is a field of research to be cultivated more or less indefinitely, like botany or chemistry, and from which a comprehensive interpretation of the modern rise of population can be expected only in the remote future if at all.

One result of this approach is the lack of a conceptual background, based on firmer evidence and more up-to-date experience, against which to judge the credibility of hypotheses which arise from individual enquiries. This has led to undue attention to small-scale studies, and opinion has veered with each additional proposal, however inconsistent with later, in some cases present-day, experience. Two examples will illustrate the consequences.

It has been suggested that in the eighteenth century inoculation against smallpox reduced mortality from the disease and may have contributed significantly to the decline of the death rate and growth of population.[11] This procedure was introduced from the Middle East in

---

[10] *Population in History, op. cit.*

[11] P. E. Razzell, 'Population change in eighteenth-century England: a reinterpretation'. *Economic History Review* (2nd series), **18** (1965), p. 312.

an attempt to prevent smallpox at a time when vaccination was un-known; it consists of inoculating, that is to say infecting, a healthy individual with material taken from a patient with smallpox. This practice appears to have been common in Britain, at least during part of the eighteenth century, but there are several reasons for question-ing its effectiveness. In the first place it assumes a substantial and pro-longed decline of the disease which cannot be confirmed from pre-registration data. Secondly, it attributes to this crude and dangerous measure, which no present day physician would have the courage or foolhardiness to use, an influence on total mortality which has not resulted, and indeed would not be expected, from any modern im-munization procedure supported by the full resources of the laboratory and by health education. And thirdly, it postulates an effectiveness which is not accepted by virologists who know smallpox, most of whom are of the opinion that inoculation is more likely to have spread than limited the infection. (Even in the eighteenth century it was recog-nized that some inoculated people suffered severe attacks which were sometimes fatal.) Indeed there could be no better illustration of the consequences of speculating without regard for up-to-date experience than the willingness of a historian to debate with a distinguished viro-logist the effects of an immunological procedure on the behaviour of a disease he probably has never seen.[12]

But there is an even more general objection to the proposals con-cerning inoculation, one which turns on an understanding of the way in which vaccination has contributed to the control of smallpox in the nineteenth and twentieth centuries. Here it is important to understand that the protection afforded by vaccination is very effective but rela-tively transitory, and it is the opinion of some of those who have had extensive experience of smallpox that we owe its control much more to surveillance and containment by vaccination of contacts with a con-firmed case rather than to mass immunization. Dixon, for example, was extremely sceptical about claims for the efficacy of the so-called mass immunization programmes, on the grounds that even if 70–80 per cent of a population has been vaccinated at some time, the majority of vaccinations are well outside the period within which protection can be considered to be effective.[13] This conclusion is supported by experi-ence in India, where smallpox remained a serious problem in spite of mass vaccination until adequate surveillance and containment were introduced. Similarly in the very successful West African programme, smallpox was eradicated, without achieving a high level of immunity in the population, by concentrating on case detection, outbreak

[12] A. W. Downie, 'Comments on "Edward Jenner: the history of a medical myth" by P. E. Razzell'. *Medical History*, **9** (1965), p. 223 (see also p. 381).

[13] C. W. Dixon, *Smallpox*. J. and A. Churchill (London, 1962), pp. 195–6, 239–48.

investigation and vaccination of contacts. And again, the 1972 Khulna epidemic in Bangladesh was brought rapidly under control through selective immunization of high risk groups; mass vaccination was not undertaken and the general level of immunity in the population is believed to have remained essentially the same.[14] In the light of this recent experience of control of smallpox, no significance can be attached to evidence that inoculation was common in the eighteenth century since, in the same circumstances, without vaccination of contacts we could not be certain of the results of the much more effective and less dangerous procedure.

Another example of erroneous conclusions which may be drawn when historical issues of this kind are considered without reference to present-day experience is provided by interpretation of the results of hospital treatment. A review of medical work during the eighteenth century suggested that hospital treatment was then ineffective, and even at times prejudicial to health, because of the risk of infecting patients at a time when the nature and means of spread of infectious diseases were unknown.[15] This conclusion was challenged, on the grounds that figures taken from the records of an eighteenth-century hospital showed that the majority of patients admitted were either cured or relieved.[16]

Those who made this suggestion were aware of some technical reasons for reservations: the hospital records do not specify patients individually and give only rounded figures for admissions and cures; and it was undoubtedly in the interest of hospitals dependent on voluntary support to present a cheerful picture of the results of their work. They were apparently unaware of a much more fundamental problem, that no present-day hospital could expect such favourable results, or could even provide records which would make it possible to assess accurately what is achieved. The significance of recent experience is so important that it will be useful to explain the reasons for these difficulties.

The patients admitted to a hospital present very different tasks. Some need only investigation of abnormal signs or symptoms, while at the other extreme patients may be admitted in coma and die without recovering consciousness. Between these examples there is a wide range of conditions which vary greatly in type, severity and duration, and their classification according to the tasks they present

[14] A. Sommer, 'The 1972 smallpox outbreak in Khulna municipality, Bangladesh: II effectiveness of surveillance and containment in urban epidemic control'. *American Journal of Epidemiology*, **99** (1974), p. 303.

[15] T. McKeown and R. G. Brown, 'Medical evidence related to English population changes in the eighteenth century'. *Population Studies*, **9** (1955), p. 119.

[16] E. Sigsworth, 'A provincial hospital in the eighteenth and early nineteenth centuries'. *Yorkshire Faculty Journal, College of General Practitioners* (June 1966), p. 24.

is an essential preliminary to assessment of the results of the work of a hospital. An acceptable classification of this kind is very difficult to achieve and is not yet available.

But even if it were possible to classify patients according to the work involved, the problem of assessing benefit within classes would remain formidable. The effectiveness of much hospital treatment is at present unknown, and there are serious ethical and technical difficulties in organizing the kinds of investigation that would be needed to assess it. However, a recent appraisal of coronary care in hospital may help to correct the impression that the outcome of treatment is in general favourable and often a cure. It was estimated that of 100 patients admitted after myocardial infarction (a heart attack) to one of the best-equipped hospitals in England, 70 would have survived without treatment, 15 would have died however treated, and the scope for benefit was restricted to the remaining 15. In the best hands, and given the requisite facilities, these 15 patients could be expected to survive; but the underlying disease conditions and the likelihood of recurrence would remain essentially unchanged. Those with experience of hospital work would be unlikely to disagree that in many other serious conditions the results of treatment are no better and the likelihood of spontaneous survival is a good deal worse. It is the patient not the doctor who talks of cures.

From a medical viewpoint the proposals concerning inoculation against smallpox and the results of eighteenth-century hospital treatment would hardly seem to require so full a discussion. However, these proposals have been taken seriously by historians, and they illustrate the pitfalls which beset eighteenth-century population study when considered without reference to present-day experience. The question remains whether the alternative approach referred to above is feasible, that is whether it is possible to by-pass some deficiencies of evidence when the modern rise of population is considered as a whole and from a background of recent knowledge.

This approach is likely to provoke objections of two kinds. One is a philosophic objection from historians, that it is misleading to attempt to understand the past in terms of the present; the other is a technical objection, perhaps mainly from demographers, that it is essential to improve the basic data and methods of analysis before relying on them to support a comprehensive hypothesis.

The first objection arises from failure to distinguish between three aspects of historical research, concerned respectively with what our predecessors were thinking, what they were doing and what they were achieving. When assessing what was thought one may indeed be misled by a present-day viewpoint, and an act of imagination is required from the historian to enable him to examine the concepts of the past on their own terms. There is no obvious reason why investigation of what our predecessors were actually doing should be prejudiced by more recent knowledge, although the latter may not in some cases be necessary. But where the purpose of research is to establish so far as possible what men were achieving, as distinct from what they thought they were achieving, then it is essential to examine their actions against the background of the most complete evidence that can be assembled. Inescapably this is the evidence available to us in the present day.

It is the last type of enquiry which arises frequently from the major issues, and particularly the medical issues, in historical demography. For example, when interpreting reasons for the decline of mortality from tuberculosis in the nineteenth century, the ideas of contemporaries about treatment are irrelevant. What is needed is a judgement of its effectiveness against the background of the vast experience of the disease now available. If we conclude, as physicians who have seriously considered the matter have concluded, that treatment of tuberculosis was ineffective before the introduction of streptomycin, there is no need for further investigation of the results of medical intervention in this disease in the nineteenth century or earlier.

The second objection – that it is essential to improve the basic data before attempting a comprehensive hypothesis – underestimates the feasibility and importance of covering the canvas, that is of considering together the main questions raised by the demography of the past three centuries. This procedure of course raises its own problems; but they are easier to recognize and more tractable than those which arise when a single issue in the eighteenth century, such as the relation between fertility and mortality or the disappearance of plague, is considered in isolation. The possibilities of the comprehensive approach can be illustrated by summarizing some conclusions which will require much fuller discussion in later chapters.

I believe it would be agreed that when the population growth of the past three centuries is considered as a whole it is essentially a declining death rate that needs to be explained. I think there is also no doubt that the trend of mortality was due predominantly to a reduction in the number of infectious deaths. Hence a central issue in historical demography is the reason for the decline of mortality from infectious diseases.

In the period since cause of death was first registered, a large majority of infectious deaths were due to the following diseases, which were also those associated mainly with the decline of mortality: tuberculosis, scarlet fever, measles, diphtheria and the intestinal infections. In all these diseases it can be said without reservation that effective immunization or therapy was unavailable before the twentieth century. We are left with one or both of the possibilities that the virulence of the organisms diminished or that there were improvements in the environment which may have reduced exposure to the diseases or strengthened the defences of those who encountered them, for example by improved nutrition.

The reduction of deaths from intestinal infections is explained largely by removal of the source of infection through improved hygiene, and from scarlet fever by a change in the virulence of the organism, the haemolytic streptococcus. In the other three diseases it is not possible to assess the precise importance of the two classes of influence (although in the case of tuberculosis there are some grounds for thinking that a substantial decline in the virulence of the tubercle bacillus is unlikely). What can be said with considerable confidence is that when these and some other infections are considered together, it is hardly credible that the enormous reduction of deaths was due to a fortuitous change in the character of the organisms which was independent of both medical intervention and environmental change. Hence, in spite of the difficulty of interpreting the trend of mortality of a disease such as whooping cough, when the infections are considered collectively there is no doubt that environmental influences played a major part in their decline.

It is on an approach of this kind that we must rely when interpreting the fall of mortality, to some extent since 1838 and still more in the pre-registration period. Indeed when considering the demography of the eighteenth century it is salutary to be reminded that it is not possible to account with certainty for the reduction of deaths from whooping cough in the present century. Still less are we likely to be able to explain the behaviour of a single disease at the earlier time when cause of death was unknown. But an interpretation of the trend of mortality since 1838 is possible without a full picture of the influences on whooping cough, and the main issues in the eighteenth century can be resolved without a convincing explanation of the disappearance of plague.

In short, the answer to the question whether it is difficult to interpret the modern rise of population is the answer Shaw gave when asked whether it is difficult to write plays: it is either easy or impossible. It is easy to establish the relative importance of changes in fertility and mortality from the time of registration of births and deaths; and, if not easy, it is not particularly difficult in the light of present knowledge to account in broad terms for the decline of the diseases which contributed to the reduction of deaths. With these issues clarified, we can turn to the uncertainties of the eighteenth and early nineteenth centuries and venture an opinion on the main questions without undue reliance on the deficient evidence available for that period. But if it is necessary to establish the basic historical 'facts of life' before attempting to formulate explanatory hypotheses[17] for the demography of the

[17] D. V. Glass, 'Introduction'. In *Population in History, op. cit.*, p. 8.

eighteenth century, then I believe an acceptable interpretation of the modern rise of population can be expected only in the distant future, if at all.

If this conclusion gives the impression that what is attempted here is a metaphysical interpretation, the treatment in the chapters which follow will I hope correct it.

2
Fertility and Mortality

Ignoring the effects of migration, an increase in the rate of population growth may be due to one or both of (a) an increase in the birth rate and (b) a reduction of the death rate. In the period since births and deaths were registered nationally in developed countries – in Sweden from 1749, in France from 1800, in England and Wales from 1838 and in most other countries somewhat later – there is no doubt about the trend of the rates; there has been a substantial reduction of mortality but no increase in birth rates which indeed, for part of the time, have declined. However, opinion is still divided about the rates in the pre-registration period, although in Sweden, where the decisive upturn in population growth was delayed until the second decade of the nineteenth century, the doubts arise in respect of at most a few years between the beginning of the modern rise of population and the registration of births and deaths. Nevertheless some historians have suggested that eighteenth-century population growth was due initially to an increase in the birth rate which resulted from withdrawal of existing restraints on fertility. This interpretation rests on the assumption that at times human populations have limited the numbers of births because of concern for the availability of food and other essentials.

At first sight it seems hardly necessary to take this suggestion very seriously, at least in the modern period. Even allowing for some reservations about the uncharted decades of the eighteenth century, it is quite inconsistent with the recorded history of technologically advanced countries. It is also out of keeping with experience of the developing world today, where those countries with some records of births, deaths and population show no evidence of effective restraints on fertility. On the contrary, such advances as have been made recently in developing countries, mainly by control of animal vectors and improved hygiene, have been offset to a considerable extent by unabated population growth. However, the proposal has been made seriously and must be taken seriously, if only because it has attractions for some historians who find it in keeping with their ideas about the relation between economic conditions and population size.

The debate is concerned broadly with two issues, the relation between fertility and mortality and identification of the common causes of death. Although these issues are related and are usually discussed together, in the present context there are some advantages in separating them. The first will be considered in this chapter and the second under diseases associated with the decline of mortality in the chapter which follows.

The relation between fertility and mortality will be examined against the background of experience of three types of populations, birds and other animals, early man and modern man.

BIRDS AND OTHER ANIMALS

Although it is doubtful whether the experience of birds and other animals has much bearing on the problems of population growth of man, particularly modern man, since this experience is sometimes cited in discussion of the rise of population it will be desirable to consider it briefly. The opinions of biologists are divided about two main issues, namely, the relation between fertility and mortality and the common causes of death in animal populations. The opposing viewpoints are presented clearly in the writings of Lack and Wynne-Edwards.

In his book *Population Studies of Birds*, Lack summarized his conclusions as follows: '(a) That the reproductive rates of birds have been evolved through natural selection and so are, in general, as rapid as the environment and the birds' capacities allow; (b) that mortality rates balance reproductive rates because bird populations are controlled by density-dependent mortality; (c) that starvation outside the breeding season is much the most important density-dependent factor in wild birds (but not necessarily in other animals); (d) that breeding pairs are dispersed broadly in relation to food supplies, through various types of behaviour which are as yet little understood but which are to be explained through natural selection.'[1] It should be noted that Lack's examples were taken mainly from birds on which his own observations were based; nevertheless he believed that his conclusions about the relation between fertility and mortality applied generally to other animals, although he recognized that the main influences on mortality were not always the same as in most wild birds.

The other viewpoint was expressed by Wynne-Edwards as follows: 'It must be highly advantageous to survival, and thus strongly favoured by selection, for animal species (1) to control their own population-

---

[1] D. Lack, *Population Studies of Birds*. Clarendon Press (Oxford, 1966), p. 280.

densities, and (2) to keep them as near as possible to the optimum level for each habitat they occupy ... Population-density must at all costs be prevented from rising to the level where food shortage begins to take a toll of the numbers – an effect that would not be felt until long after the optimum density had been exceeded. It would be bound to result in chronic over-exploitation and a spiral of diminishing returns. Food may be the *ultimate* factor, but it cannot be invoked as the *proximate* agent in chopping the numbers, without disastrous consequences.'[2]

In the present context the most important issue arising from the contrasting viewpoints quoted above is whether reproductive rates are in general unrestrained, or whether through group selection they have evolved in such a way that postnatal mortality is relatively low, because numbers born are restricted according to the resources of the environment. A decision on this issue turns largely on (a) evidence of mechanisms which effectively limit fertility and keep numbers near to an optimum, (b) the acceptability of the concept of group selection and (c) the levels of mortality which are usual among wild animals.

As examples of mechanisms limiting fertility Wynne-Edwards referred to both social behaviour which restricts reproduction in order to avoid excessive demands on food resources, and to biological mechanisms which are influenced by population density. The social behaviour includes territorial systems which limit density and reduce fertility by dispersion, and the phenomenon of social hierarchy or peck-order in birds which restricts the number of males which have access to females. Moreover he suggested that such systems have developed through selection in response not merely to the immediate food supply, but also to the potential future food supply. Biological mechanisms are said to be reduction of the number of ovulations and resorption of foetuses after conception. Other writers have included under the same heading destruction of the young after birth; but this is an example of postnatal mortality and should properly be considered among causes of death.

The objections which Lack raised to this interpretation are impressive. While agreeing that dispersive behaviour may modify population density, he suggested that it can be attributed more plausibly to natural selection than to group selection. Peck-order, he considered, has also evolved through natural selection to assist the survival of both the attacking and the retreating individuals, rather than as another means of group selection.

But perhaps the central question is whether there are grounds for accepting the concept of group selection based on restriction of group

[2] V. C. Wynne-Edwards, *Animal Dispersion in Relation to Social Behaviour*. Oliver and Boyd (Edinburgh, 1972), pp. 9 and 11.

fertility. At first sight it seems possible to believe that there are circumstances in which it is to the advantage of a group if its births are limited having regard for the resources of the environment, in which case natural selection might have led to the phenomenon of group selection. Further thought suggests that there are other examples in which it is by no means obvious that restriction of fertility would favour the group: for example a large, ill fed population exposed to an epidemic of measles might have a better chance of survival after the death of half its members than a small and better fed population in which nine tenths survived (because the disadvantages of poor nutrition might be out-weighed by the advantages of more rigorous selection of a population better able to face the hazards of the infection). This example raises the critical question of the relation between group selection and natural selection among individuals. Both concepts recognize that numbers are reduced to a level which can be supported by the resources of the environment; but under the first this is achieved mainly by limiting the number of births and under the second by postnatal mortality.

The concept of natural selection which has been extended but not changed fundamentally since the time of Darwin, implies that numbers born are greatly in excess of the numbers that can survive and that a balance between population size and resources is achieved by selective mortality. Natural selection, so conceived, favours the genotype which results in most surviving offspring in a particular environment, and thus provides a basis for adaptation to changing environments. Reduction of numbers by restriction of fertility, however, is either unselective, or is selective for genotypes which are not necessarily those best suited to the postnatal environment. (For example, selection by peck-order would not ensure that the parents are those whose offspring are best equipped genetically to meet the threat of infectious disease.) Hence while group selection might in special circumstances and for short periods be to the advantage of a population, it is difficult to accept that a mechanism which reduces capacity for adaptation by natural selection is one which operates generally in animal populations.

If such a phenomenon were widely applicable it would be expected to result in low postnatal mortality rates. Observations on birds leave no doubt that although mortality is variable and low in some species (for example in various sea birds) in many other species it is as high as 30–70 per cent per annum. Wild birds usually live only a small fraction of their potential life-span. Moreover the higher the reproductive rate the higher the annual mortality, and Lack found no evidence that reproductive rates have evolved through group selection to maintain a low level of mortality. Apart from birds, adult mortality rates in the wild appear to have been recorded for only a few mammals, fish and insects.

These observations suggest that the existence of effective restraints on fertility as a result of group selection in wild animals is far from being established. Indeed the weight of evidence is against it.

EARLY MAN

When attempting to unravel the relation between fertility and mortality, biologists and historians have turned to the experience of early man, hoping that *inter alia* it might throw some light on population growth and related issues in the more complex circumstances of modern societies. They have considered evidence mainly from two sources: first, that which can be obtained for the period when man lived as a hunter and gatherer more than 10,000 years ago; and second, observations which have been made recently on the few primitive populations which appear to be still unaffected, or little affected, by external influences. At this point I shall be concerned only with fertility and mortality, leaving to the next chapter discussion of the related problems of causes of death and standards of health in primitive people.

It should be said at once that there is no acceptable evidence about fertility and mortality in the long period before the first agricultural revolution. Since we are unable to give reliable birth rates and death rates for some countries in the world today, it is most unlikely that we shall ever be able to rely on the grossly deficient sources which are all that can be expected for early man. Some writers have concluded that fertility must have been restricted from the fact that populations were small; but the most effective means of limiting numbers to which they refer, particularly infanticide, are postnatal rather than prenatal.

A more promising source of information is a population which has retained a primitive way of life little affected by modern (including agricultural) developments. Although it is questionable whether such populations live in the same conditions as prehistoric man, useful observations have been made, for example on Indians in South America, aborigines in Australia and Eskimos in North America. However, in none of those populations has it been possible to make direct observations on fertility, and estimates have been deduced from indirect evidence. From such evidence some workers have concluded that 'primitive man seems to have curbed his intrinsic fertility to a greater extent than has the civilized world in recent centuries.'[3]

When considering this possibility it seems essential to distinguish clearly between restriction of fertility and influences on mortality. In

[3] J. V. Neel, 'Lessons from a "primitive" people'. *Science*, **170** (1970), p. 815.

discussions of population growth it is quite usual to group restraints on fertility such as prolonged lactation and abortion, with causes of post-natal death such as infanticide. In principle it might be desirable to draw the dividing line at the time of conception, and to include abortions with postnatal deaths; in practice, however, it is necessary to make the division at the time of birth, separating influences on the frequency of birth from those leading to postnatal death. On this basis the possible influences on numbers of live births are (a) re-straints on frequency of intercourse, (b) prevention of conception and (c) abortion.

The only reliable evidence of the trend of fertility of a population is the birth rate and, with one exception (Sweden), birth rates were not recorded before the nineteenth century. Even from that time, accurate assessment of the contribution of different influences, such as contracep-tion and abortion is difficult, perhaps impossible. Hence, when consider-ing whether it is likely that one or more of these influences reduced the fertility of primitive man, we are making a judgement which cannot be supported by direct evidence. Nevertheless there is a good deal of experience – experimental, clinical and epidemiological – which makes it possible to assess the possible effectiveness of these influences on the fertility of primitive people.

Even today there is no real evidence that the growth of any human population has been limited substantially by restraints on the frequency of intercourse. As the world's literature amply attests, the urge to copulate is so strong that it has led men to lie, steal, rape, kill, go to war and burn 'the topless towers of Ilium'. This is not to ignore taboos on intercourse, or to suggest that social conventions in respect of customs such as age at marriage have no effect on fertility. But there are no grounds for believing that such practices effectively limit popula-tion size, and there must be few people who think that the formidable problem of population growth in developing countries today can be solved by appeals for continence. It seems very unlikely that in primi-tive man the sexual urge was weaker or social restraints more effective.

There are many different kinds of influences which may affect the likelihood of conception after intercourse. One class comprises the stresses imposed by the external environment, of which the most important is undoubtedly deficient food. Both experimental and clinical evidence suggest that the effect of such deficiencies is felt first on the newborn (leading to sickness or death), next on the probability of conception (through interruption of the sexual cycle) and last on the pregnancy itself. Hence when a population is exposed to restriction of food, increased postnatal mortality is more conspicuous than effects on the frequency or outcome of pregnancy. Nevertheless there is reason to believe that the effects of insufficient food on fertility are profound. It has been shown recently that in young women in developed countries a minimum weight for height is necessary both for the menarche and for maintenance of the menstrual cycle, and relatively modest weight losses result in amenorrhoea.[4] This suggests that in developing countries today, among women not using contraceptives the number of pregnancies is probably limited more by lack of food than by practices such as prolonged lactation (discussed below). It also seems likely that poor nutrition was an important cause of infertility in early populations. However, an uncontrolled external influence of this kind has little bearing on the question whether early man deliberately 'curbed his intrinsic fertility'.

A more relevant example is the frequently cited effect of prolonged lactation, which is said to be common among primitive people. From experimental work on rats and mice it is clear that it is the stimulus of suckling rather than lactation which interrupts the cycle, and this effect can be demonstrated in non-pregnant animals. But suckling does not postpone the cycle indefinitely, and even while the stimulus is vigorously maintained, the cycle returns and pregnancy occurs when the females are exposed to males.[5] Human observations also indicate that the effectiveness of prolonged lactation on reducing fertility has been overestimated. For example, 30 per cent of a group of postpartum women became pregnant within a year after delivery; two fifths of them were still lactating at the time of conception and one tenth conceived without having menstruated.[6] In another study, the cycle reappeared within five months of birth in 40 per cent of women whose children were wholly breast fed. It was concluded that in women, as in most experimental animals, the cycle is fairly effectively suppressed during the early months of lactation; it reappears in an increasing proportion of women as lactation proceeds and returns more rapidly if the child is partially weaned.[7] Moreover, the capacity of the breast to secrete enough milk to feed a child diminishes after the early months, and children who are kept at the breast for the prolonged periods quoted for primitive people must be receiving their food largely from other sources. Under such conditions the stimulus of suckling is reduced and the effect on fertility must be small.

The other possible influences on conception are contraceptive

[4] R. E. Frisch and R. Revelle, 'Height and weight at menarche and a hypothesis of menarche'. *Archives of Disease in Childhood*, **46** (1971), p. 695. R. E. Frisch and J. W. McArthur, 'Prediction of minimum weights for menarche and the restriction of menstrual cycles'. In press.

[5] H. Selye and T. McKeown, 'Production of pseudo-pregnancy by mechanical stimulation of the nipples'. *Proceedings of the Society of Experimental Biology*, **31** (1934), p. 683.

[6] C. G. Peckham, 'An investigation of some effects of pregnancy noted six weeks and one year after delivery'. *Bulletin, Johns Hopkins Hospital*, **54** (1934), p. 186.

[7] T. McKeown and J. R. Gibson, 'A note on menstruation and conception during lactation'. *Journal of Obstetrics and Gynaecology of the British Empire*, **61** (1954), p. 824.

measures of the kinds which have become common in the modern world. There is little evidence of the practice of birth control in the English demographic literature of the century preceding the Industrial Revolution[8] and, while individuals and groups have undoubtedly avoided pregnancy by *coitus interruptus* and other methods, the earliest indication that they did so on a scale which affected national fertility trends is the decline of the French birth rate from the end of the eighteenth century. It is instructive that this occurred first in a Catholic country and in spite of severe religious taboos on contraceptive measures.

The third of the major influences on fertility is termination of an established pregnancy by abortion. As recent experience in Japan and Britain shows, there is no doubt about the effectiveness of this procedure and the only question is whether it was feasible with the knowledge and techniques available to early man. There is no reason to think so. In spite of the extensive lore about the effects of influences such as drugs, violence and psychological stress, it is difficult to interrupt a normal pregnancy by any means other than direct interference with the contents of the uterus. This intervention can be undertaken with reasonable success and safety during the first sixteen weeks of pregnancy by an experienced doctor operating under appropriate conditions. In any other circumstances intervention is both unreliable and dangerous, and often results in the septic abortions which were common before the grounds for legal abortion were liberalized. It seems hardly credible that abortion can have provided for early man what it has not until recently provided for modern man, an effective means of restraining fertility.

There is little doubt about the frequent use, and no doubt about the effectiveness of the other method of limiting population size usually discussed in this context, namely the deliberate killing of infants and children after birth. However, this is an aspect of mortality and should properly be considered with other causes of postnatal death rather than as a means of reducing fertility. Here we are concerned only with the general conclusion that there is no direct evidence about the fertility of early man, and examination of the possible means of limiting the number of births – by abstaining from intercourse, by contraception or by abortion – suggests that they are very unlikely to have been effective. The more convincing reason for slow population growth is a high level of mortality.

---

[8] R. R. Kuczynski, 'British demographers' opinions on fertility, 1600–1760'. In *Political Arithmetic*, edited by L. Hogben (London, 1938), p. 283.

MODERN MAN: DEVELOPED COUNTRIES

Although it has seemed desirable to consider wild animal populations and primitive man (mainly because their experience is sometimes cited in this context) it is questionable whether they have much relevance to interpretation of population growth in modern man. Those who believe that our early ancestors effectively restrained their fertility have had to recognize that this ability has been lost, for there is no evidence of it in developing countries today. The explanation usually suggested is that the ecological balance which formerly existed has been disturbed, and this disturbance is said to date from the time when man abandoned his nomadic life as a hunter and gatherer. Clearly the populations which expanded in the eighteenth century were far removed from the primitive way of life in which ecological equilibrium is said to have existed. Hence the modern growth of population should be interpreted on the available evidence, and without undue reliance on experience of other animals or primitive peoples.

A newcomer to the demography of the past three centuries might easily conclude that the central question is whether the initial spurt in the rate of population growth in the eighteenth century was due to an increase in the birth rate or a decrease in the death rate. A considerable literature is concerned with this issue; there have been numerous studies of local sources such as parish registers which attempt to establish the trend of fertility and mortality in the pre-registration period; and the writings of economic historians, particularly those concerned with the relation between population growth and economic and industrial development, appear to assign a central place to the birth rate/death rate controversy.

However, there are grounds for thinking that the importance of this issue is somewhat exaggerated, particularly in relation to interpretation of the modern rise of population as a whole. In the first place, the period in which there is any serious doubt about the behaviour of the rates – that is the interval between the beginning of the modern rise and national registration of births and deaths – is not long. In England and Wales it may be as much as a hundred years before registration in 1838; but in France it extended only to 1800, and in Sweden it can have been no more than a few decades before 1749. Thus if we look at the trend of fertility and mortality in Europe as a whole, the uncertainty arises only in respect of quite a short period before the mid eighteenth century.

Another reason for thinking that this issue has had undue prominence is that changes in birth rate and death rate are less significant than the question: What disturbed either rate? For whether the aim is interpretation of the modern rise of population or an understanding of the relation between population size and economic conditions, the main requirement is assessment of the various influences – agricultural, industrial, medical, etc. – which may have contributed to the growth of population. In this task, appraisal of the behaviour of birth rate and death rate is only a means to the end. For if we conclude that the birth rate increased we have then to consider why it did so; and if we believe mortality declined we must investigate the reasons for the reduction of deaths from the diseases chiefly concerned. Of course when the eighteenth century is considered on its own, as it usually is in historical demography, it seems essential to come to a conclusion about the trend of fertility and mortality as a preliminary to further enquiry. But when the eighteenth century is approached against a background of conclusions concerning the post-registration period, it may be possible to examine the major issues without first having resolved the birth rate/death rate controversy. For example, to anticipate the fuller discussion of these matters in later chapters, if the growth of population before the twentieth century cannot be attributed to a decline of mortality which was due to a change in the character of infectious diseases or to immunization and therapy, we must conclude that it resulted from improvement in the environment, whether this led to a reduction of mortality or an increase in fertility. In this approach the latter remains an interesting and, in some respects, an important issue; but it hardly deserves the central place in historical demography that it has been assigned hitherto.

With due regard for these reservations it will nevertheless be desirable to discuss the behaviour of the birth rate and death rate in the eighteenth century, if only to see more clearly the limits of our knowledge. Again the approach depends on whether we think this problem is best attacked directly or, as I suggested in the opening chapter, in the light of conclusions concerning the post-registration period. It will therefore be necessary to examine birth rates and death rates from the times when they were first recorded reliably. This examination will be based on four countries in Western Europe – England and Wales, Sweden, France and Ireland.

The post-registration period
Figures 2.1 and 2.2 give the birth rates and death rates of the four countries from the times when they were first recorded nationally. They provide no evidence that the rates have increased; indeed for most of the time they have been falling. The relation between fertility, mortality and population growth is shown for each of the countries separately in figures 2.3–2.6.

In England and Wales (figure 2.3) the birth rate began to fall in 1871–80; the increase during the period 1841–50 is usually attributed

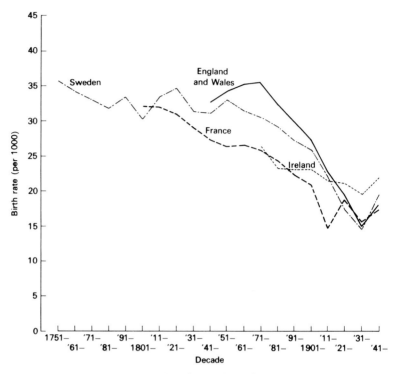

2.1 Birth rates from the times when first registered.

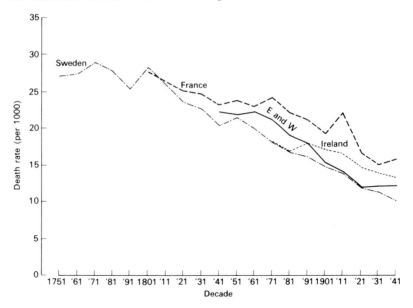

2.2 Death rates from the times when first registered.

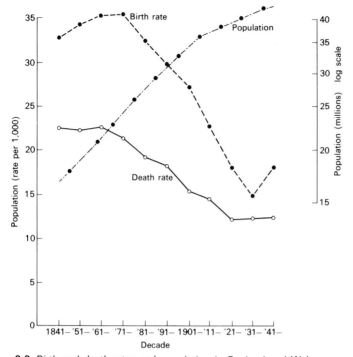

2.3 Birth and death rates and population in England and Wales.

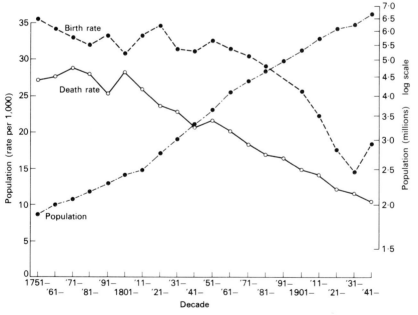

2.4 Birth and death rates and population in Sweden.

to deficient registration in the early years. The death rate was fairly constant for the two decades after registration but fell from 1861–70.

The Swedish data (figure 2.4) are of particular interest, since they are available from 1751. During the second half of the eighteenth century the birth rate and death rate were high and fluctuating, the birth rate being generally above 30 (per 1000 population) and the death rate above 25, rates similar to those estimated for England and Wales in the same period. The death rate began to fall during the early nineteenth century while the birth rate continued at about the eighteenth-century level until the third quarter when it also declined.

The contribution of the birth rate and death rate to the early growth of the Swedish population can be estimated as follows. The population increased by 28 per cent between 1761–5 and 1801–10 and by 54 per cent between 1811–15 and 1856–60. For the two fifty-year periods mean birth rates were the same (32·6) and mean death rates 27·6 and 22·7 respectively. Thus the increase of the population between 1750 and 1850 was due to a reduction of mortality; the increase during the second half of the ighteenth century, when mortality remained more or less constant, is attributable to an excess of births over deaths established by the middle of the century. For the whole period 1751–1800 the birth rate was 33·6 and the death rate 27·4.

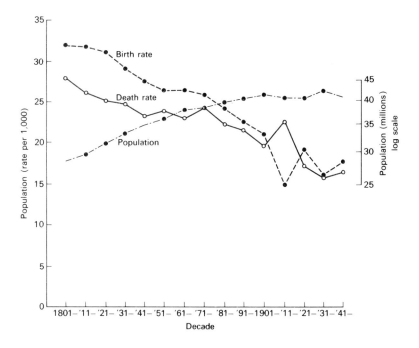

2.5 Birth and death rates and population in France.

In France (figure 2.5) the death rate declined from 1800 until the middle of the century; it then remained fairly constant until about 1875 when it declined again. The rate in France was in general somewhat higher than in England and Wales, 24 and 22 respectively in about 1850. However, the most remarkable difference between the two countries was in the behaviour of the birth rate, which fell in France almost continuously from 1800, at least seventy years before the beginning of the decline in England and Wales. At the middle of the nineteenth century the birth rates in France and England and Wales were 27 and 34 respectively.

In Ireland (figure 2.6) because of the deficiencies in the data no confident conclusion can be drawn about the behaviour of the birth rate and death rate before 1871, except that a considerable excess of births over deaths had been established by that time. There was a reduction in the birth rate during the last three decades of the nineteenth century, when the death rate remained more or less constant. However, a substantial excess of births over deaths remained, and indeed throughout the period 1871 to 1950 the decline in the birth rate and the decline in the death rate were remarkably similar.

Considered as a whole, the data for these four countries since registra-

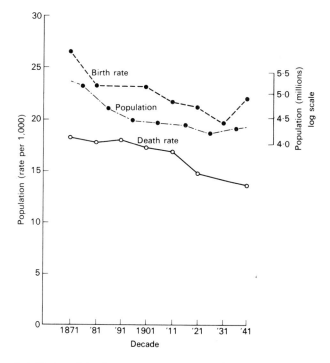

2.6 Birth and death rates and population in Ireland.

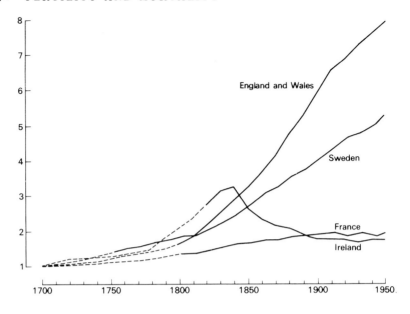

2.7 Sizes of populations relative to their sizes in 1700.

tion provide no evidence of rising birth rates, but show that the growth of population was due to an excess of births over deaths established before registration and to a subsequent decline of mortality. This leaves unexplained the reason for the excess of births over deaths already established at the time of registration; but before considering the pre-registration period we must examine briefly the effects of migration, which are known to be substantial in several countries and profound in Ireland, where population size is lower today than it was in the mid nineteenth century.[9]

One of the most remarkable features of the demographic history of Europe is the variation between countries in rates of population growth. Figure 2.7 shows relative growth rates in the four countries between 1700, for which the estimated populations are taken as 1, and 1950. In this period the population increased 8·0 times in England and Wales, 5·3 times in Sweden, 2·0 in France and 1·7 times in Ireland.

In assessing the reasons for these differences it is essential to consider the effects of migration. They can be estimated by comparing the actual rates of population growth with those that would have resulted if population size were determined only by birth rates and death rates with no losses or increases from migration. These estimates can of course

[9] This examination is based on the analysis by T. McKeown, R. G. Brown and R. G. Record in 'An interpretation of the modern rise of population in Europe'. *Population Studies*, **27** (1972), p. 345.

be made only from the time when births and deaths were first recorded: 1841, when Sweden and France are compared with England and Wales, and 1871, in the case of Ireland. While these dates are relatively late in the history of the modern rise of population, they include the periods when emigration was most important.

In Sweden, from 1841, elimination of the effects of migration substantially increases the estimate of population, whereas in England and Wales there is only a small difference between the calculated and actual numbers. Indeed the *calculated* rates of population growth are very similar in Sweden and England and Wales, so that the difference between the *actual* rates in this period was determined almost entirely by emigration from Sweden. However, emigration was not significant before 1860, so that some other explanation must be sought for the slower expansion of the Swedish population before this time. The explanation is probably to be found in the lower Swedish birth rate.

The rate of population growth was slower in France than in England and Wales from 1800 and the two rates had diverged considerably by 1841, when birth and death rates became available for both countries. It is therefore possible to investigate the effects of migration on only part of the large difference in rates of population increase which occurred between 1800 and 1950. The slower growth of the population of France between 1841 and 1951 is not explained by emigration. Indeed, throughout the period the increase was greater for the actual than for the calculated population, which indicates that migration resulted in a net increase. The explanation of the difference in growth rates between France and England and Wales must therefore be sought in the behaviour of the birth rate and death rate. Both contributed to the difference. From 1841 to 1950, except for a short time, the birth rate was lower in France than in England and Wales and the death rate was considerably higher. Over most of the period the influence of the lower birth rate was somewhat greater than that of the higher death rate.

Although it is not possible to assess the effect of emigration from Ireland by the method described above before 1871, when births and deaths were first registered, its earlier influence on population size is evident (figure 2.7). The population of Ireland was increasing at about the same rate as that of England and Wales during most of the first half of the nineteenth century. Large-scale emigration began in the fifth decade and from that time population size fell sharply. Comparison between the actual rate of population growth in Ireland from 1871 to 1950 and the rate which would have resulted if population size had been determined solely by the numbers of births and deaths, shows that emigration was the main, although not the only, reason for the difference in population growth rates of Ireland and England and Wales.

The respective contributions of birth and death rates to the difference can also be estimated. From 1871 to 1911 approximately, the birth rate was considerably higher in England and Wales than in Ireland and this was the main reason for the residual difference in rates of population growth over that period, that is for that part of the total difference which was not due to emigration from Ireland. From 1931 the birth rate was lower in England and Wales and from this time until 1950 the rate of increase of the calculated populations was a little greater in Ireland than in England and Wales. The contribution of death rate differences over the whole period 1871 to 1950 was relatively small.

I can now summarize conclusions concerning the contribution of births and deaths to the increase of population in the period since both were registered nationally. In the four countries considered, the growth of population was due to an excess of births over deaths established by the time of registration and to a subsequent decline of mortality. The much lower rates of population growth in the three other countries than in England and Wales are attributable mainly to emigration, in the case of Ireland and Sweden, and to a lower birth rate, in the case of France. At least from the time of registration, it is the decline of mortality that needs to be explained in order to account for the growth of population.

The eighteenth and early nineteenth centuries
In the light of this conclusion the pre-registration period will be approached as follows. Since registration – 1749 in Sweden, 1800 in France and 1838 in England – there is no evidence of increasing birth rates; on the contrary over most of the period birth rates and death rates have declined. However, an excess of births over deaths had been established in the three countries by the times of registration, and we must consider whether this was due to a previous increase in the birth rate or to a decline of mortality. It should be noted that in the case of Sweden the question is only whether the trend of the birth rate and death rate in the few decades preceding the mid eighteenth century was quite different from that in the two and a half centuries which followed.

Until recently there were few serious doubts about the answer to this question, at least in England where it was generally accepted that the increase of population was due to a fall in the death rate brought about by advances in medicine. This interpretation was based largely on the work of Griffith, whose book *Population Problems of the Age of Malthus* was published in 1926.[10] Griffith examined medical developments in the eighteenth century – expansion of hospital, dispensary and midwifery services, changes in medical education, advances in physiology and morbid anatomy, and introduction of inoculation against smallpox –

---

[10] G. T. Griffith, *Population Problems of the Age of Malthus*. Second edition, Frank Cass (London, 1967).

and concluded that they led to a substantial decline in mortality. It was not until a quarter of a century later that this interpretation was questioned seriously, by Habakkuk[11] who doubted the efficacy of the measures referred to, and by McKeown and Brown[12] who considered the major developments – in surgery, midwifery, medicines, hospitals, etc. – and came to the conclusion that they did not lead to a reduction of the death rate. Since that time the question concerning the influence of the birth rate and death rate on eighteenth-century population growth has again been raised, and opinion is still divided between those who believe mortality declined (hence the interest in such matters as the results of eighteenth-century hospital work and the practice of inoculation against smallpox) and those, particularly among economic historians, who have examined once again the possibility that fertility increased in response to improved economic conditions.

In the opening chapter it was noted that no statistics are available which put this issue beyond dispute, and interpretation is inevitably influenced by the point of view from which it is approached. Griffith, for example, was convinced that medical effort had a substantial effect on the death rate, while Habakkuk and others were impressed by the apparent significance of the birth rate in pre-industrial societies. Before considering once again the uncertainties of eighteenth-century evidence, we should recognize that the probable influence of the rates is determined mainly by their levels. When birth rates and death rates are high the population is more likely to increase by a reduction of the death rate than by an increase in the birth rate. When the rates are low the reverse is true.

When death rates are high, as in developing countries today and in all countries in the recent past, mortality is due largely to a high incidence of infectious diseases. The level of infection is determined mainly by the standard of living, and even modest improvements are reflected rapidly in a lower death rate. This reduction affects mainly children and infants; unless offset by a decline in fertility it results first, in an increase in population, second, in a temporary reduction in the birth rate (because the number of persons alive is increased but not at once, proportionately, the number of births), and third, in a rise in the birth rate, as young people who have survived reach reproductive age. Hence when the death rate is high, relatively small improvements in the standard of living are reflected immediately in an increase of population and, possibly later, in a rise in the birth rate.

It is much more difficult to effect an increase in population by a

[11] H. J. Habakkuk, 'English population in the eighteenth century'. *Economic History Review* (2nd series), **6** (1953), p. 117.

[12] T. McKeown and R. G. Brown, 'Medical evidence related to English population changes in the eighteenth century'. *Population Studies*, **9** (1955), p. 119.

primary increase in the birth rate when that rate is already high. Natural fertility sets limits to the number of children born, and unless the rate of reproduction has previously been restricted (for example by contraception or changes in frequency or age of marriage) it cannot be increased much. That is to say, when the birth rate is high it is unlikely to increase further except as a result of a shift in the age distribution of the population, secondary to reduced mortality.

When both rates are low population size is more likely to be influenced by a higher birth rate than by lower mortality. The low birth rate is restricted voluntarily, and might be increased, for example in response to improved economic conditions. But lack of medical knowledge sets limits to the extent to which mortality can be reduced, even among people in the most favourable circumstances. For example, inspection of the causes of stillbirth and infant deaths indicates that without new knowledge perinatal mortality is unlikely to fall much below the best levels already achieved in favoured sections of the populations of some developed countries. And where expectation of life is already high we cannot expect a substantial extension of life of persons in the older age groups.

There is little doubt that both rates were high in the eighteenth century. The birth rate fluctuated between 30 and 35 in Sweden between 1751 and 1801 and it was at about the same level in France and England at the times of registration (1801 and 1838 respectively). The death rates were somewhat lower, between 25 and 30 in Sweden and France and between 20 and 25 at the later date in England. Estimates which have been made for the pre-registration period, for example, by Brownlee and Griffith for England, are consistent with these figures and in some cases are higher. It is against this background that we must enquire whether the excess of births over deaths established by the time of registration was due to an increase of the birth rate or a decrease of the death rate.

The birth rate in a given year is determined by the proportion of the population which consists of women of childbearing age, and the number of children born during the year to such women.

The proportion of the female population which consists of women of childbearing age may increase as a result of an increase in the birth rate, or of a change (increase or decrease) in mortality rates which favours females in or below the reproductive age groups more than those in older age groups. Because of high early mortality and the marked association between mortality rates and family size (see table 2.1), an increase in the birth rate would need to be very substantial to have much influence on the age distribution of the female population when mortality from infection is high, unless accompanied by a reduction in mortality rates. If this is true a substantial increase in the proportion of females in reproductive age groups is unlikely to have occurred except as a secondary effect of a change in mortality.

Ignoring variation in the incidence of illegitimacy, the number of children born to women of childbearing age is determined by (a) the proportion of women who marry, (b) mean age of women at marriage, (c) reproductive capacity of married women and (d) the extent of deliberate limitation of family size.

(a) It is recognized that there is an association between economic circumstances and marriage rates. Data for England and Wales examined by Glass show a high correlation ($r = 0 \cdot 706 \pm 0 \cdot 065$) between marriage rates and an index of real wages during the period 1856–1932.[13] But the correlation is determined mainly by changes in age at marriage, rather than by variation in the proportion of women who ultimately marry. This is suggested by the fact that between 1851 and 1911 the percentage of persons married varied between 19 (1911) and 28 (1871) for ages 20–24, but remained fairly constant at 86–8 for ages 50–54. From 1851, from which time data are fairly complete, a woman's chance of getting married before the age of 50 fluctuated between 82 per cent (in 1910–12) and 96 (in 1940). Since the proportion of women who can marry is considerably below 100 per cent (it is well below 96 per cent for any prolonged period) because of the greater proportion of women than of men in the adult population, it is clear that at no time since 1851 has there been scope for a substantial increase. There is no evidence that frequency of marriage was substantially lower in the eighteenth century. Data examined by Griffith[14] and Marshall[15] show no considerable increase in English marriage rates during the second half of the century; reliable statistics are not available for the first half.

(b) We should require very strong evidence before accepting that changes in age at marriage had a substantial influence on the mean number of children born to women of childbearing age during the eighteenth century. As suggested above the correlation between marriage rates and economic conditions is probably attributable to variation in age at marriage, rather than to changes in the proportions who ultimately marry. But it does not follow that variation in age at marriage was substantial, for the high correlations are quite compatible with relatively small changes in mean age. For example in England and Wales for the years 1890–1907 and 1926–32, correlations between marriage rate and an index of real wages were 0·603 and 0·677 respec-

[13] D. V. Glass, 'Marriage frequency and economic fluctuations in England and Wales, 1851 to 1934.' In *Political Arithmetic, op. cit.*, p. 266.
[14] *Population Problems of the Age of Malthus, op. cit.*, p. 34.
[15] T. H. Marshall, 'The population problem during the Industrial Revolution'. *Economic Journal* (1929), p. 444.

tively; yet changes in mean age at marriage of women during the period 1896 to 1951 were small.

Moreover, there are reasons for believing that postponement of marriage would have less influence on the number of live births than is commonly supposed. In the first place there is no evidence that within fairly wide limits age of husband has any considerable influence on reproductive capacity, and when they postpone marriage men frequently marry women younger than themselves. In England and Wales in 1911, when postponement is believed to have been common, men at all ages over 21 married younger wives and the difference in mean age increased as age at marriage increased: mean ages of wives of men aged 22 and 35–9 were 21·98 and 31·97 respectively. In Ireland, where postponement of marriage is common, it is also more marked among men than among women: in 1936 proportions unmarried in the age group 35–9 were 48·4 per cent and 32·8 per cent for males and females respectively. Secondly, in the absence of widespread birth control, a moderate increase in mean age at marriage would not have a very marked effect on fertility. For women married 30–35 years in rural Ireland in 1911, whose ages at marriage were under 20, 20–24, 25–9 and 30–34, mean numbers of live births were 8·81, 8·04, 6·79 and 5·57 respectively. The impression that fertility drops sharply with increasing age derives from consideration of the general population of women, who marry relatively early. In these circumstances, mothers who have a first child late have smaller families than those who have a first child early, partly because the remaining reproductive period is shorter, and partly because the birth of a first child at a late age means that on the average they are less fertile. The comparison provides no reliable information about the number of children to be expected when women of normal fertility postpone reproduction. The best indication of the effect of postponement of childbirth among normal women is obtained by relating mean numbers of liveborn children to age at marriage (as above), or by examining the proportion of women who were childless according to age at marriage.

In short, if we may accept the Irish data as a rough guide to the effect of postponement of marriage on the number of liveborn children in families whose size is not intentionally restricted, an advance in mean age of wives at marriage of about 5 years would be needed to reduce the mean number of live births by 1. Since 1896 variation in mean age of women at marriage in England and Wales has not been large (range: 24·66–27·14). Unless changes in age at marriage in the eighteenth century were of quite a different order, it seems unlikely that they can have had a very marked influence on the average number of live births in a family.

(c) A third influence affecting the number of children born to women of childbearing age is reproductive capacity, and it has been suggested that it may have fluctuated during the eighteenth century as a result of disease, changes of diet and other environmental influences. This possibility cannot be excluded. But the effect of such influences on reproductive capacity – defined as the ability to conceive and give birth to living children – were probably small as compared with their effect on mortality in infancy.

(d) The methods of limiting family size which might have been effective during the eighteenth century were abstinence, abortion and *coitus interruptus*. Needless to say we have no worthwhile information about them. Abstinence was recommended by Malthus and others as the only acceptable means of avoiding pregnancy, but it is doubtful whether it has ever had much influence on population trends. Effective and safe methods of abortion were not available until recently. Moreover, the probability of death of the child after birth must have made termination of unwanted pregnancies less urgent than it is today. *Coitus interruptus* is among the oldest forms of contraception; it is less reliable than many other methods, and to be effective requires more self-control than is usually credited to the majority of people. Nevertheless the early fall in the French birth rate is usually attributed to withdrawal. As already noted, Kuczynski found little evidence of the practice of birth control in the English demographic literature of the century preceding the Industrial Revolution.

This examination of possible causes of a change in the birth rate suggests that an increase is unlikely to have occurred during the eighteenth century, except as a secondary result of a reduction of mortality. Moreover, the effect of an increase in the birth rate on population would be seriously reduced by postnatal mortality. Infant mortality (deaths in the first year of life) can hardly have been less than 200 per 1000 live births (the rate was 150 in 1900), and may have been considerably more. The extent of mortality in childhood is exhibited in table 2.1, which gives numbers of previous live births and surviving children for 1389 pregnant women attending the Westminster Dispensary between 1774 and 1781. However large the number of previous live births, the mean number of surviving children is in no case higher than 3.38.

The data also show an association between the proportion of surviving children and parity and, while this association is, of course, considerably influenced by the different periods at risk (children in 9-child families had a much longer period at risk than children in 1-child families), mortality was evidently affected by family size. For example, in families with 9–10 previous children, 2 in 3 died within a few years of birth. It can scarcely be doubted that this death rate was much higher than the average for all children. In this case, the influence of a rise in the birth rate on population would have been largely offset by a secondary rise in mortality (because the additional children would be added mainly to existing families).

If the primary cause of the rise of population is unlikely to have been an increase in the birth rate, is it more reasonable to attribute it to a change in the death rates? The view that mortality declined in England during the later years of the eighteenth century is widely accepted; what has been questioned is the conclusion that this was the primary cause of the increase of population rather than a secondary result of changes in the age composition of the population brought about by a rising birth rate in earlier decades. Two points have a bearing on this issue.

Table 2.1 Mortality according to parity (from data for the Westminster General Dispensary, 1774–81, reported by Bland, 1781)[16]

Parity (number of previous children)	Number of women (a)	Total number of children born (b)	Total number of children living (c)	Proportion of children surviving (c)/(b)	Mean number of children surviving (c)/(a)
1–2	553	807	430	0·53	0·78
3–4	377	1300	592	0·46	1·57
5–6	227	1224	502	0·41	2·21
7–8	130	966	364	0·38	2·80
9–10	55	517	177	0·34	3·22
11–24	47	605	159	0·26	3·38
Total	1389	5419	2224	0·41	1·60

In the first place, experience in the nineteenth and twentieth centuries, including that of developing countries today, leaves no doubt that the high level of mortality in the eighteenth and earlier centuries was due predominantly to infectious disease. Moreover, mortality was much greater in infancy and childhood than in adult life. Brownlee[17] estimated mortality in London during the first two years of life to be 300–400 (per 1000 live births) and according to Edmonds[18] half the infants baptized in London in the period 1770–89 were dead before the age of 5. The association between mortality and age was examined by Bland who concluded that for women attending the Westminster Dispensary between 1774 and 1781, 5 of 12 children born were dead before the age of 2 and 7 of 10 before the age of 16.[19] His estimate is based on the erroneous premise that mortality and frequency of births are unrelated to family size; nevertheless it is clear that mortality was

[16] R. Bland, 'Some calculations ... from the Midwifery Reports of the Westminster General Dispensary'. *Transactions of the Royal Society*, **71** (1781), p. 366.

[17] J. R. Brownlee, 'The health of London in the eighteenth century'. *Proceedings of the Royal Society of Medicine*, **18** (1925), p. 75.

[18] T. R. Edmonds, 'On the mortality of infants in London'. *Lancet*, **1** (1835), p. 692.

[19] 'Some calculations ...', *op. cit.*, p. 369.

highest soon after birth. The same conclusion emerges from Brownlee's data. In these circumstances there is no doubt that any significant improvements in way of life would have led to a reduction. Hence if there were advances in standard of living in the eighteenth century, they would have had more effect on population growth by reducing the death rate than by increasing the birth rate.

Secondly, Swedish data referred to above show that in the country where births and deaths were first registered, from the mid-eighteenth century the growth of population was due to a decline of mortality. The same is true of other countries whose birth and death rates were recorded from the first half of the nineteenth century or earlier. Without exception they show no evidence of increasing birth rates; on the contrary, over most of the post-registration period both birth rates and death rates have declined. We should need strong evidence for believing that something quite different occurred in the earlier period.

In conclusion, three observations are important to assessment of the behaviour of the birth rate and death rate in the eighteenth century: according to modern standards mortality was very high; the high death rates were due mainly to infectious disease; and the greatest risks were experienced by infants and young children. The level of the birth rate is less significant, although in general it also was undoubtedly high.

Of the possible causes of an increase in the birth rate, only a change in age at marriage requires serious consideration. The effect of postponement of marriage on fertility is probably less than has been thought, because when men delay marriage they usually marry women younger than themselves (in this context age of husband has no independent significance), and the decline in fertility with increasing age of wife is smaller than is commonly supposed. A change in mean age of marriage during the eighteenth century is unlikely to have been great enough to have had a substantial effect on the birth rate. But perhaps more important, so long as mortality from infection remained high, a rise in the birth rate would have had relatively little effect on population growth, because a high proportion of children would die soon after birth. The proportion dying would be greater than the prevailing mortality rates suggest, because the additional children would be added chiefly to existing families. Mortality increases sharply with increasing family size.

Under the conditions described, the fall in the death rate could have been due to a reduction in deaths from infectious disease, even in the absence of a specific medical contribution. Moreover, a primary reduction in mortality from infection would have had a profound effect on population growth, both because the reduction is greatest in young age groups, where expectation of life is longest, and because a rise in the birth rate is a possible secondary result.

MODERN MAN: DEVELOPING COUNTRIES

If there is an analogue to the pre-industrial societies of the eighteenth century, it is to be found not in wild animals or early man, but in the populations of the so-called developing countries of today. Most of them have not yet experienced any considerable amount of industrialization, although like eighteenth-century Britain and France they are far removed from the ecological equilibrium which is said to have existed before the first agricultural revolution. They have also been affected in various ways by the coexistence of countries at an advanced stage of technological development and a remote village, such as Lalibella in Ethiopia, which still retains a primitive, if not a 'natural' way of life, may have become accustomed to the daily arrival of a DC3 and, if the tourist traffic flourishes as its sponsors hope, may well in time have its Hilton. If there is evidence that the pre-industrial societies of the recent past had effective restraints on fertility which under favourable conditions might be released, it is in the developing countries of today that we might expect to find this.

There is no such evidence. In some countries data concerning fertility and mortality are either unavailable or unreliable. Where figures have been published they show that these countries have consistently high birth rates, in many cases twice as high as those of the more advanced countries. Comparison of death rates is of limited value, since in view of the large age variation the rates need to be corrected for age differences before they can be compared. Infant mortality rates (deaths of liveborn children in the first year of life) are more meaningful, and those countries which have high infant mortality rates, without exception, have very high birth rates. For example in the data published by the World Health Organization the figures for countries with infant mortality rates higher than 100 (per 1000 live births) in 1970 were as follows:[20]

	Birth rate (per 1000 population)	Infant mortality rate (per 1000 live births)
Egypt	34·9	116·3
Liberia	50·9	137·3
South Africa (coloured population)	36·8	132·6
Haiti	37·3	146·5

There are undoubtedly other populations with equally high rates which are not shown, or are inaccurately entered, in the United Nations publication. (For example, the birth rates of the rural populations of

[20] World Health Statistics Annual (1970), volume 1. World Health Organization (Geneva, 1973), pp. 10, 11.

many countries of Latin America are over 40.) But these figures are sufficient to show, what is indeed not seriously questioned, that present-day developing countries have very high birth rates and, during the period in which they have been observed, provide no evidence of effective restraints on fertility.

To summarize: national statistics for several European countries leave no doubt that the growth of population since births and deaths were first registered was due to an excess of births over deaths established by the time of registration and to a subsequent decline of mortality. Before registration the birth rate and death rate were unknown; but in Sweden, where they were recorded from the mid-eighteenth century, the period of uncertainty is at most a few decades. For that time, when both rates were undoubtedly high, a reduction of mortality is a more credible explanation for the growth of population than an increase of fertility. But whatever doubts there may be about the first half of the eighteenth century, when the modern rise of population is considered as a whole it is clearly a substantial reduction of mortality that has to be explained.

3
Diseases which declined

In interpretations of population growth, consideration of the relation between fertility and mortality is usually linked with appraisal of the causes of postnatal death. This practice was introduced by Malthus, whose conclusions were summarized on the first page of his *Essay on the Principle of Population*: 'The tendency of all animated life is to increase beyond the nourishment provided for it.' This is a compressed statement which implies two propositions: numbers born are greater than numbers that can survive; and the level of mortality is determined by the availability of food. To the present day these themes are associated in discussion, and they probably require to be associated in the interpretation outlined by Wynne-Edwards.[1] For the suggestion that populations achieve an optimum breeding rate adjusted according to the resources of the habitat needs to be examined in relation not only to the habitat but also to the common causes of death (since it implies that the level of mortality is not determined substantially by lack of food). However, since I have concluded that the modern rise of population was due to a decline of mortality rather than to a removal of restraints on fertility, the reasons for the decline can be considered in their own right and quite separately from the trend of fertility. This is the approach which will be taken in this chapter. Again, as in the preceding one, I shall examine briefly the experience of other animals and early man before turning to the influences on mortality during the past three centuries.

BIRDS AND OTHER ANIMALS

In general, knowledge of the level of mortality must precede information about cause of death; for while it might be thought possible to investigate the causes of mortality before its frequency, in practice it

[1] V. C. Wynne-Edwards, *Animal Dispersion in Relation to Social Behaviour*. Oliver and Boyd (Edinburgh, 1972).

is easier to count births and deaths than to obtain a reliable assessment of cause of deaths. Since adult mortality rates in the wild have been measured only for some birds, a few mammals, fish and insects, it is clear that the common causes of death for most animals in their natural habitats are unknown. Nevertheless a good deal of evidence has been obtained about a number of species, particularly birds, and it is on this that any general conclusions must largely rest.

The common causes of death in wild animals are predation, disease and starvation, to which must be added in the case of certain species, destruction by man. In most bird species examined by Lack, predation, disease and human destruction were unimportant and he concluded that 'food shortage was probably the main density-dependent mortality factor'.[2] However, he recognized that this was not necessarily the order of importance of the major influences in other animals: 'The number of most birds, carnivorous mammals, certain rodents, large fish where not fished and a few insects are limited by food . . . the number of gallinaceous birds, deer and phytophagous insects for at least most of the time are limited by predators (including insect parasites).' In this interpretation food supplies are considered to set an upper limit to the growth of populations, but in some animals this limit is not reached because of high mortality from other causes.

Having regard to the enormous importance of disease, and particularly infectious disease, as a cause of premature death in human populations, it is interesting that it appears to be relatively uncommon in those species of wild animals that have been examined. The explanation is probably that many animals do not achieve the population densities which are required for the survival and spread of microorganisms, although some, particularly insects, undoubtedly do.

EARLY MAN

In the previous chapter I concluded that it is very unlikely that early man was able to limit his fertility effectively, and that the more acceptable explanation of the slow growth of population in the long period before the first agricultural revolution is a high level of mortality. It should be noted that this conclusion was drawn, not from information on birth rates of primitive people, which is not available, but from assessment, against the background of present-day knowledge, of the feasibility of control of births by continence, contraception and abortion. The question remains of the common causes of mortality, particularly those which are believed to be predominant in other animals – starvation, disease and predation. And since man, uniquely among

[2] D. Lack, *Population Studies of Birds*. Clarendon Press (Oxford, 1966), pp. 276, 287.

living things, has been more successful at defending himself against other animals than against his own species, homicide (including infanticide) and war are much more significant than predation.

There are two lines of approach which have led to the idea that early man enjoyed a healthy life in ecological balance with his environment. One is from interest in the requirements for health of modern man, and it has brought recognition that in important ways he has departed from the conditions of life under which man developed. The cardio-vascular system evolved when physical exercise was inescapable and the digestive system when plant foods contained a substantial proportion of fibre. There is reason to believe that a good deal of ill health today is due to the change from a 'natural' way of life, and it seems an attractive corollary that when living under primitive conditions, early man was in general healthy.

The same conclusion has been drawn from a few examinations of primitive peoples who have survived to the present day. Some, though by no means all, are said to be quite healthy, at least until they acquire infections from visiting investigators; and this observation might be thought to be confirmed by the remarkable athletes who have descended from the African highlands to win some of the most coveted prizes in competitive sport. The widespread ill health in developing countries of Asia, Africa and Latin America appears to be inconsistent, but those who believe that early man was healthy attribute this anomaly to the fact that these populations have lost the advantages of one way of life without gaining those of the other; that is to say they have neither the natural conditions of early man nor the hygiene, medical care and secure food supply of modern man.

However, these conclusions need to be examined closely, since at first sight the idea that early man was healthy seems to be out of keeping with the belief that mortality was high and life expectation low. For it has generally been agreed by those who have studied primitive peoples that mortality rates are high, even if not so high as in some developing countries today, and that old people are relatively uncommon.[3] It is of course not inconceivable that in such a population death by killing or accident might keep numbers at or below the level at which the resources of the habitat would maintain them in health. But this means either that the restraints on fertility are inadequate, since postnatal deaths are also required to limit numbers; or that numbers killed are excessive having regard to the resources of the environment.

Before considering briefly the causes of death I should like to emphasize two points made in a recent discussion of health and disease

[3] J. V. Neel, 'Lessons from a "primitive" people'. *Science*, **170** (1970), p. 815.

in hunter-gatherers.[4] The first refers to the deficiencies of evidence: 'Hunters today do not live in wholly aboriginal or "prehistoric" states of health, and historic or ethnographic records offer little data upon which to base speculations about prehistoric conditions of health.' Any assessment of the health of primitive people must therefore be influenced profoundly by our general understanding of the major causes of mortality in modern as well as early man. The second point concerns the great variability of experience among primitive peoples, 'the fallacy in generalizing about "hunter-gatherers" as though they were some kind of homogeneous cultural-genetic ecological unity. They are diverse, their hunting territories are diverse and so are their diseases and ways of life.' The question must be asked whether, having regard for the lack of evidence and variation of circumstances, it is possible to make any generalization about the causes of death during man's evolution. With some reservations, I believe it is possible.

The causes of death can be divided broadly into two classes according to whether man was or was not directly responsible for them. The first class comprises the various forms of homicide, including infanticide, sacrifice, cannibalism, geronticide and war. It is generally accepted that these deaths were common, and the rate of infanticide alone, which no doubt varied widely, has been estimated as between 15 and 50 per cent of all births.[5] At such levels infanticide would be sufficient to account for a high level of mortality and would provide a considerable restraint on the growth of population. Langer's historical review suggests that infanticide was practised widely both in ancient and modern times, and even today may be relatively common.[6] Some years ago in a developing country I attended three seminars concerned with the health problems of families. The numbers of surviving children in the families considered were 19 boys and 2 girls. This remarkable sex ratio was probably due to a high level of female infanticide which passed, I may say, without comment.

Among causes of death for which man was not directly responsible, the important ones are starvation and disease, particularly infectious disease. Some, although by no means all, of those who have examined the experience of primitive people have concluded that they were reasonably well fed and that sickness and death from food deficiency were uncommon. Again the evidence is inadequate; but with due regard for the undoubted variation at different periods and in different

[4] F. L. Dunn, 'Health and disease in hunter-gatherers'. In *Man the Hunter*, edited by R. B. Lee and I. Devore, Aldine Press (Chicago, 1972), p. 228.
[5] R. E. Lee and I. Devore, 'Problems in the study of hunters and gatherers'. In *Man the Hunter, op. cit.*, p. 11.
[6] W. L. Langer, 'Infanticide: a historical survey'. *History of Childhood Quarterly*, **1** (1974), p. 353.

regions of the world, it is hard to believe that food supplies have not always been a serious problem for man, and that deficiencies were not frequent and at times disastrous. To think otherwise is to conclude that the famines which have been recorded throughout history to the present day did not occur or were unusual in the prehistoric period before man learned to cultivate plants and animals. It seems unlikely that primitive man, living a nomadic life, was able not only to control his numbers according to the resources of the environment, but also to handle his casual food sources and storage in such a way that he was protected from the effects of climate and season.

These accomplishments, if they existed, have clearly been lost, for the rural populations of large areas of Africa, Asia and Latin America not only have insufficient food, but lack the knowledge which would make it possible to get the full benefit from the foods that are available. Kwashiokor is a result of ignorance as well as of poverty. It has of course been suggested that the skills of early man were lost through contact with more developed societies, and it is not difficult to believe that this is true for the unfortunate rural people who have made their homes in or near the major cities of developing countries. (The problem was possibly seen in its most acute form in Calcutta after the partition of India and Pakistan.) It is not so easy to see why it should be true for the rural populations who still cultivate indigenous foods and prepare them in traditional ways, little influenced by modern refinements. Indeed there is evidence that under such conditions African populations, for example, do not have the disease pattern of western countries, although they soon acquire it when they move to the west or come under its influence, particularly in respect of diet. Nevertheless these present-day rural people do suffer from the effects of insufficient food, sometimes manifested by deficiency diseases and frank starvation, but more frequently appearing in the form of endemic infectious diseases associated with malnutrition. It is difficult to see why, in the transition from a nomadic to a more settled but still primitive rural life, the knowledge which would have made it possible to avoid the effects of food shortage should have been lost.

Early man's experience of infectious disease will be considered in chapter 4. Here it should be said that although the nature and frequency of his infections are of course unknown, there are grounds for thinking that some of them at least were less common than in later pre-industrial societies, and possibly than in developed countries today. This suggestion is based on the observation that populations of a considerable size are needed to maintain specifically human infections (such as measles, smallpox and mumps) which can survive only by rapid transmission from one host to another. Populations of the requisite size and in close contact did not exist before the first agricultural revolution, although whether this means that infectious disease due to micro-organisms specifically adapted to the human species was almost nonexistent, as suggested by Burnet, is still a debated issue.[7] Our information about the other diseases and disabilities of early man is equally scanty, although it seems reasonable to believe that gatherers and hunters were prone to injury. It is more difficult to accept that injuries (including those caused by predators) were the main causes of ill health and death.[8]

In conclusion, reliable evidence concerning health and disease in early man is scanty. The belief that mortality rates were high rests partly on present-day observations of primitive people, but still more on recognition that postnatal mortality is a more credible explanation for the slow growth of population than the possible methods of restraint on fertility (continence, contraception or abortion). It is generally accepted that death in infancy and childhood, particularly from infanticide, was common and that alone would account for a high level of mortality.

The causes of mortality fall broadly into two classes, the first comprising those for which man was responsible (all forms of homicide, including war) and the second, those for which he was not directly responsible, namely food deficiencies, disease (particularly infectious disease) and injury arising from hunting and gathering. On the evidence available, or likely to become available, it is impossible to assess the relative contributions of these influences, which no doubt varied from one population to another and from time to time. What can be said is that all these causes are related to the environment, and particularly to its food supplies. For if homicide in its various forms was common, this was presumably determined ultimately by limitations of resources. And if starvation or infectious disease associated with food deficiency were important, they resulted even more directly from lack of food.

Viewed in this way, the common causes of death in early man were analogous to those outlined by Lack in his interpretation of the experience of wild animals.[9] In some animals food shortage is the main 'mortality factor'; in others food supplies set an ultimate limit to the growth of population, but the limit is not always reached because of other influences such as predation. With due regard for the deficient evidence and variable conditions, the experience of early man can be interpreted broadly in the same terms. At some times the level of mortality was probably determined mainly by shortage of food and associated disease; at other times the food limits may not have been reached because of a high death rate from causes such as infanticide and tribal war. The relative importance of these two kinds of influences undoubtedly varied from time to time and between populations. This

[7] F. M. Burnet, *Virus as Organism*. Harvard University Press (Cambridge, 1946), pp. 30–31.
[8] S. Boyden, 'Evolution and health'. *Ecologist*, **3** (1973).
[9] *Population Studies of Birds, op. cit.*

is consistent with the conclusion that the main restraint on population growth was a high level of mortality determined directly or indirectly by the availability of food.

Assessment of reasons for the reduction of mortality since the eighteenth century requires identification of the diseases associated with the decline. The discussion will be based mainly on data for England and Wales; and it will be desirable to consider in turn the post-registration period, when cause of death was certified, and the pre-registration period, for which national data are not available.

The Post-registration Period

Cause of death has been registered in England and Wales since 1837, and it might be thought that whatever the difficulties before that time it would be relatively easy to follow the subsequent trend of mortality attributed to specific diseases. Problems arise both from vagueness and inaccuracy of diagnosis and from changes in nomenclature and classification. For example, there must be doubts about the diagnosis of tuberculosis at a time when it was not possible to x-ray the chest or identify the tubercle bacillus. In the Registrar General's classification scarlet fever was not separated from diphtheria until 1855, nor typhus from typhoid before 1869. Even the less exacting task, so important for the present discussion, of distinguishing infectious from non-infectious causes of death, presents difficulties. For example, deaths attributed to diseases of the heart and nervous system included a considerable but unknown number due to infections such as syphilis. These problems will be considered later in relation to the decline of mortality from individual diseases.

In spite of the difficulties, several attempts have been made to assess the diseases which contributed to the decline of mortality during the nineteenth and twentieth centuries. Longstaff examined the trend between 1861–70 and 1876–80 and later extended the examination to 1888.[10] He concluded that the decrease of deaths was due mainly to reduced mortality from typhus and tuberculosis and, to a lesser extent, from scarlet fever, smallpox, diarrhoeal diseases, diphtheria and measles. Phillips conducted a similar enquiry for the period 1851 to 1905 and again underlined the diminished mortality from typhus, smallpox, whooping cough, typhoid, scarlet fever, tuberculosis and diphtheria.[11]

[10] G. B. Longstaff, 'The recent decline in the English death rate considered in connection with the cause of death'. *Journal of the Statistical Society*, **47** (1884), p. 221.

[11] S. Phillips, 'A review of mortality statistics during the last half century'. *Clinical Journal*, **30** (1908), pp. 55 and 73.

In an address to the Royal Statistical Society, Greenwood examined English death rates from 1841–5 to 1926–30 and suggested some reasons for their decline.[12] Stocks reviewed experience in the first half of this century.[13] However, the most comprehensive examination was that of Logan, who considered in some detail the changes in causes of death between 1847 and 1947.[14]

It is no criticism of these papers to say that their main concern was to examine the decline of mortality rather than the reasons for it, and that when interpretation was attempted it was written in very general terms, in which the contribution of different influences was not considered. Logan's conclusions are characteristic of the approach:

> The reduction or elimination of some of the infectious diseases can be related directly to definite preventive measures such as vaccination (smallpox), immunization (diphtheria) and improved sanitation (cholera and typhoid). The prevalence or the fatality of other diseases have declined because of less specific measures associated with a higher standard of living – better food, clothing and housing, purer air, earlier and fuller medical attention. Special *ad hoc* public health services, maternity and child welfare, venereal disease and tuberculosis clinics and the like, have reduced the risk of death among certain groups. The medical inspection of schoolchildren prevents serious defects remaining undetected and untreated. In industry special hazards have been recognized and the workers protected; conditions in workshops and in factories have been improved and the hours of work reduced. In parallel with these preventive measures there have been great advances in curative medicine and surgery.

But although these reports have differed from this book both in their aims and in the periods covered, they leave no doubt about the predominant contribution of the infectious diseases to the decline of mortality.

Figure 3.1 shows the trend of the death rate for males and females from 1841 to 1971. For the nineteenth century the rates for the six decades were standardized to correspond to the age of the population of 1901; for the twentieth century the rates are for the first year of each decade, again standardized in relation to the 1901 population. Standardization is needed to correct for the changing age structure since, with an ageing population, the crude (i.e. unstandardized) death rates

[12] M. Greenwood, 'English death rates, past, present and future'. *Journal of the Royal Statistical Society*, **99** (1936), p. 674.

[13] P. Stocks, 'Fifty years of progress as shown by vital statistics'. *British Medical Journal*, **1** (1950), p. 54.

[14] W. P. D. Logan, 'Mortality in England and Wales from 1848 to 1947'. *Population Studies*, **4** (1950), p. 132.

understate the fall of mortality which actually occurred. Throughout the period death rates were consistently higher for males than for females. They began to fall in the eighth decade of the nineteenth century and the decline has continued to the present day.

But although the death rates for the whole population changed little before 1871–9, in some ages (2–24) the decline began somewhat earlier.[15] During the nineteenth century the fall of mortality was proportionately greatest at those ages (2–34) at which mortality was lowest

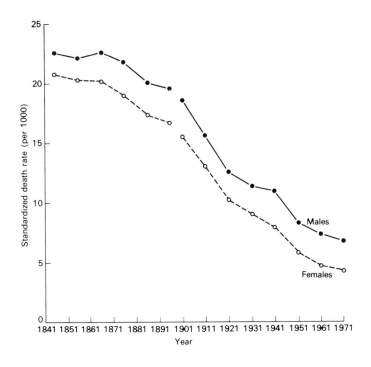

3.1 Death rates in England and Wales.

in 1841–9; there was no improvement in infant mortality (deaths in the first year of life) or in mortality at ages over 45.

From 1901, the rates of decline were marked at ages under 45, considerable for females between 45 and 74, and relatively small for males over 45 and for females over 75. In general the trend of mortality by age is similar to that which began in the late nineteenth century, but there were two exceptions: the rapid reduction of deaths in the first year of life from 1900; and the fall in middle and late life, especi-

[15] T. McKeown, R. G. Record and R. D. Turner, 'An interpretation of the decline of mortality in England and Wales during the twentieth century'. *Population Studies*, **29** (1975), p. 391.

ally in females. These improvements at the beginning and towards the end of life are the most important ways in which mortality experience has changed since the turn of the century.

Assessment of the contribution made by different diseases to the decline of mortality is based on data published in the *Annual Reports of the Registrar General*. The chief difficulty in interpretation arises from uncertainty about the reliability of death certification; it is particularly serious in the nineteenth century when understanding of the nature of infectious disease was revolutionized by the work of bacteriologists. Nevertheless the significance of this work to diagnosis, from the first decades after registration when little was known to the end of the century when a good deal was known, is not so great as might be thought. Many of the infections were fairly clearly identified on clinical grounds, and medical experience of them was much greater than it is today.

In the discussion which follows a broad distinction will be made between conditions attributable to micro-organisms and conditions which are not. This distinction cannot be made in all cases. For example, in the immediate post-registration period rheumatic heart disease was not separated in national statistics from other diseases of the heart. Hence, although rheumatic heart disease is attributable to streptococcal infection, it is included here with other diseases of the heart among conditions not associated with micro-organisms. In the early period nephritis was classified with dropsy which is partly non-infective in origin, so again, when data for the mid-nineteenth century are used, nephritis is included with conditions not attributable to micro-organisms, although most cases are the result of bacterial infection. There are a few other infective conditions which even today cannot be separated in national statistics; for example, congenital malformations which result from rubella. With these reservations, the broad distinction between infective and other conditions can be made with reasonable confidence.

Conditions attributable to micro-organisms will be subdivided further into three groups – airborne, water- and food-borne, and other. This division, according to mode of transmission of the organisms, is essential for the examination of reasons for the decline of mortality in later chapters.

Table 3.1 shows the trend of mortality from diseases in these groups between 1848–54 and 1971. The years 1848–54 have been taken to represent the beginning of the post-registration period because certification of cause of death was incomplete during part of the first decade after registration. The death rates for 1848–54 and for 1971 were standardized to correspond with the age distribution of the 1901 population.

Table 3.1 Death rates* (per million) in 1848–54, 1901 and 1971

	1848–54	1901	1971	Percentage of reduction (1848–54 to 1971) attributable to each category	For each category, percentage of reduction (1848–54 to 1971) which occurred before 1901.
I Conditions attributable to micro-organisms:					
1 Airborne diseases	7259	5122	619	40	32
2 Water- and food-borne diseases	3562	1931	35	21	46
3 Other conditions	2144	1415	60	13	35
Total	12965	8468	714	74	37
II Conditions not attributable to micro-organisms	8891	8490	4070	26	10
All diseases	21856	16958	5384	100	30

* Standardized to the age/sex distribution of the 1901 population

Table 3.2 Standardized death rates (per million) from airborne diseases

	1848–54	1901	1971	Percentage of reduction from all causes (1848–54 to 1971), attributable to each disease	For each disease, percentage of reduction (1848–54 to 1971) which occurred before 1901
Tuberculosis (respiratory)	2901	1268	13	17·5	57
Bronchitis, pneumonia, influenza	2239	2747	603	9·9	Increase
Whooping cough	423	312	1	2·6	26
Measles	342	278	0	2·1	19
Scarlet fever and diphtheria	1016	407	0	6·2	60
Smallpox	263	10	0	1·6	96
Infections of ear, pharynx, larynx	75	100	2	0·4	Increase
Total	7259	5122	619	40·3	32

Of the fall of mortality which occurred between 1848–54 and 1971, three quarters were associated with conditions attributable to micro-organisms and one quarter with non-infective conditions. Forty per cent of the reduction was due to airborne diseases, 21 per cent to water- and food-borne diseases and 13 per cent to other infections.

The table also shows (in the last column) the proportion of the decline between 1848–54 and 1971 which occurred by the turn of the century. It was 30 per cent for all diseases, 37 per cent for the infections and 10 per cent for conditions not attributable to micro-organisms.

This result is at slight variance with the conclusion of McKeown and Record that the decline of mortality during the nineteenth century was due wholly to a reduction of deaths from infectious diseases.[16] The difference is accounted for partly by the fact that the earlier analysis was concerned mainly with the specific communicable diseases and did not include bronchitis and pneumonia among the infections. (Deaths from these diseases increased during the nineteenth century and so offset a slight decrease of deaths from conditions not due to micro-organisms.) But the difference is also related to the change in the period examined (1851–60 to 1801–1900 in the earlier publication, and 1848–54 to 1901 in the present analysis).

Airborne diseases As noted above, two fifths of the reduction of the death rate was associated with airborne diseases and about a third of this improvement occurred before 1901 (table 3.1). Difficulties which arise in identification of the individual diseases have also been mentioned, particularly the grouping of diphtheria with scarlet fever until 1855. Before this year deaths from croup were shown separately, and while this term undoubtedly included other infections, since it probably comprised mainly laryngeal diphtheria it has been accepted in the diphtheria and scarlet fever group.

Table 3.2 shows the contribution made by different airborne diseases to the total decline of mortality between 1848–54 and 1971. Respiratory tuberculosis accounted for 17·5 per cent of the reduction, and more than half of this improvement (57 per cent) occurred before the end of the nineteenth century. Mortality from the disease fell continuously, at least from the time when cause of death was first registered, and by the fifth decade it had fallen by about one quarter.

The next largest contribution was from bronchitis, pneumonia and influenza (9·9 per cent). It is unfortunately necessary to group these conditions together because there is some evidence of transfers from

---

[16] T. McKeown and R. G. Record, 'Reasons for the decline of mortality in England and Wales during the nineteenth century'. *Population Studies*, **16** (1962), p. 94.

one category to another. For example, both pneumonia and bronchitis deaths show an increase in years of high influenza prevalence, and it seems clear that a number of influenza deaths were ascribed wrongly to pneumonia, and, even more frequently, to bronchitis. Confusion between bronchitis and pneumonia, at least in old people, is suggested by the fact that the death rate of men aged 75 and over attributed to pneumonia increased by 9·2 per 1000 between 1901 and 1971, whereas deaths from bronchitis decreased by 5·5 per 1000 in the same period. It is also possible that some deaths which earlier would have been certified as 'old age' were transferred to this category. If this is so, the number of deaths from these respiratory diseases would have been larger in 1901 and the decline by 1971 correspondingly greater. As shown in table 3.2, deaths from these diseases increased between 1848–1854 and 1901 but fell between 1901 and 1971. The trend of mortality will be examined more closely later, but here it should be said that there is evidence that the reduction of the death rate from pneumonia, bronchitis and influenza began before the end of the nineteenth century. This was the conclusion reached about pneumonia by Magill, who stated in the presidential address to the American Association of Immunologists in 1954 that 'the rapid decline of pneumonia death-rates began in New York State before the turn of the century and many years before the "miracle" drugs were known.'[17]

Diphtheria and scarlet fever together were associated with 6·2 per cent of the fall of mortality (from 1848–54 to 1971) and 60 per cent of this reduction occurred before 1901. It is of course possible to consider the diseases separately after 1855, and McKeown and Record showed that the death rate from scarlet fever fell rapidly in the second half of the nineteenth century, whereas that from diphtheria increased slightly.[18] Since 1901 both have declined, and there have been very few deaths from either disease in England and Wales since 1951.

Whooping cough contributed 2·6 per cent to the reduction of mortality. The fall of the death rate was relatively small in the nineteenth century, and accounted for only about a quarter of the decrease between 1848–54 and 1971. Nevertheless mortality from the disease has declined almost continuously since about 1870, and there are now few deaths in England and Wales (26 in 1971, of which 22 were in children under 1 year).

Measles was associated with 2·1 per cent of the fall of the death rate between 1848–54 and 1971. During the nineteenth and early twentieth centuries childhood mortality from measles was relatively high, but it fell rapidly from about the time of the First World War. Nevertheless

[17] T. P. Magill, 'The immunologist and the evil spirits'. *Journal of Immunology*, **74** (1955), p. 1.
[18] 'Reasons for the decline of mortality', *op. cit.*

Table 3.3 Standardized death rates (per million) from water- and food-borne diseases

	1848–54	1901	1971	Percentage of reduction from all causes (1848–54 to 1971), attributable to each disease	For each disease, percentage of reduction (1848–54 to 1971) which occurred before 1901
Cholera, diarrhoea, dysentery	1819	1232	33	10·8	33
Tuberculosis (non-respiratory)	753	544	2	4·6	28
Typhoid, typhus	990	155	0	6·0	84
Total	3562	1931	35	21·4	46

measles remains an important infectious disease; in 1971, 135,000 cases were notified in England and Wales and there were 28 deaths.

Smallpox contributed 1·6 per cent to the total reduction of the death rate and most of this improvement (96 per cent) occurred before 1901. Since about 1910 there have been relatively few deaths from smallpox in the British Isles.

It seems unnecessary to comment in detail on the remaining infections (of the ear, pharynx and larynx), since together they accounted for only 0·4 per cent of the fall of mortality. There are also some airborne diseases which, because they caused few deaths and had little influence on the trend of the death rate, have been classified under 'other conditions'.

Water- and food-borne diseases   The decline of mortality associated with water- and food-borne diseases is shown in table 3.3. Together they were responsible for approximately a fifth of the fall of the death rate between 1848–54 and 1971 and nearly half (46 per cent) of the improvement occurred before 1901.

It seems desirable to group together the diarrhoeal diseases. In the twentieth century they comprised essentially diarrhoea, dysentery and enteritis; but in the period 1848–54 there was also a considerable number of deaths attributed to cholera which are therefore included under the same heading. These diarrhoeal diseases were responsible for about a tenth (10.8 per cent) of the total fall in mortality before 1971. One third of this decline occurred before 1901.

The deaths associated with non-respiratory tuberculosis in 1848–54 (table 3.3) are those shown in the Registrar General's classification as scrofula, tabes mesenterica and hydrocephalus. The deaths attributed to hydrocephalus include some due to the congenital and other forms of the disease; however, in the nineteenth century the majority of deaths were undoubtedly from tuberculous meningitis, and since the different types were not then separated in national statistics, it seems right to classify them with other forms of non-respiratory tuberculosis. This overstatement of non-respiratory tuberculosis deaths is compensated by the inevitable omission of deaths due to renal and bone and joint tuberculosis. From 1901 the classification was reasonably comprehensive, and there is little difficulty in following the trend of mortality from that time. The disease was responsible for 4·6 per cent of the reduction of the death rate between 1848–54 and 1971 and 28 per cent of the improvement occurred before 1901.

Since typhus was not distinguished from typhoid fever before 1869, they are classified together in table 3.3. It is unfortunate that this grouping is necessary, since typhus is not spread by water and food and should properly be included under the third category of 'other

Table 3.4 Standardized death rates (per million) for other diseases attributable to micro-organisms

	1848–54	1901	1971	Percentage of reduction from all causes (1848–54 to 1971), attributable to each disease	For each disease, percentage of reduction (1848–54 to 1971) which occurred before 1901.
Convulsions, teething	1322	643	0	8·0	51
Syphilis	50	164	0	0·3	Increase
Appendicitis, peritonitis	75	86	7	0·4	Increase
Puerperal fever	62	64	1	0·4	Increase
Other infections	635	458	52	3·5	30
Total	2144	1415	60	12·6	35

conditions'. The balance of deaths due to typhus and typhoid before 1869 is uncertain, but from that time at least the latter greatly outnumbered the former. The death rate from typhus fell rapidly in the last decade of the nineteenth century and there have been few deaths from the disease during the twentieth. Together these diseases were associated with 6 per cent of the reduction of mortality between 1848–1854 and 1971 and 84 per cent of the decline occurred before 1901. It is worth underlining the fact that the rate of decline of mortality before the turn of the century was much greater for the enteric diseases, then spread mainly by water, than for the diarrhoeal diseases spread mainly by food.

Other diseases due to micro-organisms There remains for consideration a miscellaneous group of conditions of infective origin, which are not spread mainly by air, water or food, or for which the certification of cause of death was unsatisfactory (as in the case of 'convulsions and teething'). Together the diseases of this class were responsible for 12·6 per cent of the total reduction of mortality between 1848–54 and 1971 and 35 per cent of this decrease occurred before 1901.

Table 3.4 shows the contribution made by different conditions; the largest (8 per cent) was from convulsions and teething. Although these terms were long regarded as unsatisfactory, they were employed in 1901 when 20,956 deaths were attributed to them. By 1911 the term 'teething' was no longer accepted, although it was still used in association with convulsions. The use of convulsions also diminished; only 9 deaths were so certified in 1961 and none in 1971. This reduction was presumably due mainly to transfer of deaths to other and more acceptable causes, as well as to the general decline of the underlying infections.

Most of these deaths were infective. They were associated particularly with diseases of childhood (whooping cough, measles, otitis media, meningitis, pneumonia, gastroenteritis, etc.), and in this analysis attention has been restricted to deaths under five years in the Registrar General's reports, excluding the small number at later ages. Although it is not possible to identify the true causes of death included under convulsions and teething, it is probable that most of them were airborne infections.

The other diseases specified in table 3.4 contributed little to the total decline of mortality: syphilis, 0·4 per cent; appendicitis and peritonitis, 0·4 per cent; and puerperal fever, 0·4 per cent. Except in the case of appendicitis there are no special difficulties in identifying these conditions in the Registrar General's classification. Syphilis is interpreted here to include the principal manifestations of the disease – general paralysis of the insane, locomotor ataxia and aneurism. Until

62

Table 3.5 Standardized death rates (per million) from conditions not attributable to micro-organisms

	1848–54	1901	1971	Percentage of reduction from all causes (1848–54 to 1971), attributable to each condition	For each condition, percentage of reduction (1848–54 to 1971) which occurred before 1901
Congenital defects	28	126	127	0·6 increase	Increase
Prematurity, immaturity, other diseases of infancy	1221	1249	192	6·2	Increase
Cerebrovascular disease	890	803	603	1·7	30
Rheumatic heart disease	64	487	88	0·1 increase	Increase
Other cardiovascular disease	634	1186	1688	6·4 increase	Increase
Cancer	307	844	1169	5·2 increase	Increase
Other diseases of digestive system	706	586	105	3·6	20
Other diseases of nervous system	316	305	63	1·5	4
Nephritis	615	391	46	3·5	39
Other diseases of urinary system	107	91	23	0·5	19
Pregnancy and childbirth (excluding sepsis)	130	71	3	0·8	46
Violence	761	640	345	2·5	29
Old age	1447	930	16	8·7	36
Other diseases	1665	781	202	8·9	60
Total	8891	8490	4670	25·6	10

1951 the frequency of deaths from cardiovascular syphilis was slightly understated, because the classification did not separate those due to syphilitic valvular disease. Until 1931 the number of deaths attributed to puerperal fever was also somewhat reduced because infective deaths associated with abortion were not identified.

Conditions not attributable to micro-organisms The conditions included under this heading are shown in table 3.5. They are a heterogeneous collection, having in common only that they are not due to micro-organisms or, in a few cases which are, that they cannot be identified in national statistics. Together these conditions were associated with 25·6 per cent of the total decline of mortality since 1848–54 and 10 per cent of this reduction occurred before 1901.

There are many problems of terminology and classification. For example, the term 'old age' was common, and although it was recognized to be unsatisfactory more than a fifth of the deaths of persons aged 65 and over were attributed to it in 1901. From 1911 the use of the term diminished, deaths presumably being transferred to more acceptable causes of death, both infectious (for example pneumonia) and non-infectious (heart disease). This is the background of a category of deaths which contributed 8·7 per cent to the total decline.

The heading 'prematurity, immaturity and other diseases of infancy', associated with 6·2 per cent of the decline, undoubtedly covers a large number of very different conditions. (It excludes congenital defects.) As knowledge of neonatal diseases increased, the classification was expanded, and some deaths were transferred to more satisfactory categories. However, these distinctions cannot be made in the nineteenth and early twentieth centuries, so it is necessary to combine prematurity with other diseases of infancy. It should be emphasized that deaths in this class increased in the late nineteenth century, and did not fall until after 1901. This largely explains the observation that the decline of infant mortality was delayed until after 1901.

Difficulties arise with 'other diseases of the nervous system'. For example, poliomyelitis was not specified in the 1901 and 1911 classifications, and was probably grouped with 'diseases of the cord' (which therefore include a few deaths of infective origin). However, this error is probably small, for poliomyelitis was not then or later a common cause of death. Paralysis agitans did not appear in 1901 and 1911, but has been included since 1921 although some cases are believed to result from virus infection. This may be true also of multiple sclerosis, shown separately from 1921.

These examples, which could be extended, are characteristic of the problems of terminology and classification which arise with conditions not attributable to micro-organisms. There is a further difficulty. In the case of the infections the division according to mode of transmission will facilitate the later interpretation of reasons for their decline. No such approach is possible in the case of non-infectious causes of death. For example, cancer mortality has increased during this century. This increase is mainly the result of deaths from lung cancer caused by smoking, and it has masked a fall in mortality from some other cancers, brought about by therapy and, no doubt, other influences. The picture is also complex in cardiovascular disease, where a large increase in deaths from myocardial infarction may have obscured a reduction of deaths from other forms. Violence also should be mentioned, since the contribution of treatment is probably understated by an increase in the frequency of severe injuries.

It should be noted that the reduction of mortality was lower for males than for females (21·3 per cent and 31·6 per cent respectively in the twentieth century). This sex difference is due largely to the increase in male deaths from lung cancer and cardiovascular disease, without which the fall in male mortality from non-infectious deaths would have been much greater. This means that the decline of male mortality for non-smokers during this century has been considerably greater than these figures suggest.

Eighteenth and early nineteenth centuries
In chapter 1 I suggested that we cannot rely on estimates of birth rate, death rate and cause of death before 1838 when national statistics were not recorded. Nevertheless in order to interpret the rise of population in the eighteenth and early nineteenth centuries one must come to a conclusion about three issues: the respective contributions of a fall of the death rate and rise of the birth rate to the growth of population; the extent of the decline of mortality; and, at least in broad terms (such as infective and non-infective), the types of death which declined. The first of these issues was discussed in chapter 2, and I concluded that the main reason for the rise of population was a substantial reduction of the death rate. The remainder of this discussion is therefore concerned with an appraisal of the extent of this reduction and the causes of death associated with it. The conclusions will draw on experience in the post-registration period.

Table 3.1 gave the standardized death rates per million for the three periods 1848–54, 1901 and 1971. In order to set in perspective the extent of the decline of mortality which occurred before and after registration, an estimate is needed for the death rate at the beginning of the eighteenth century. The Swedish death rate for the period 1751 to 1800 was 27·4, and the rate for England and Wales is believed to have been at about the same level or a little higher. With due regard for the lack of direct evidence it is therefore suggested that at the

Table 3.6   Reduction of mortality since 1700

	Death rates (per million)	Reduction of mortality	Percent in each period of total reduction	Percent of reduction in each period attributable to infections
1700	30000			
		8144	33	100*
1848–54	21856			
		4898	20	92
1901	16958			
		11574	47	73
1971	5384			
1700–1971		24616	100	86

*This estimate does not allow for the probable contribution of infanticide and starvation, discussed in the text

beginning of the eighteenth century the death rate in England and Wales was about 30. On this assumption the proportion of the reduction of mortality which has occurred since 1700 is shown in table 3.6 for three periods: 1700 to 1848–54 (33 per cent); 1848–54 to 1901 (20 per cent); 1901 to 1971 (47 per cent).

These estimates are of course based on an assumption about the death rate in 1700 which cannot be confirmed. But it would probably be agreed that the rate is unlikely to have been lower than that of Sweden in the second half of the eighteenth century (27·4), or, in the light of the death rates in several countries at the time of registration (figure 2.1), higher than 35. At various levels within these limits, the proportion of the decline of the death rate between 1700 and 1971 which occurred in the pre-registration period would have been as follows:

Death rate in 1700	Percentage of the decline in the pre-registration period
27·4	25
30·0	33
32·0	38
35·0	44

A choice between these estimates cannot be made confidently, but it is not critical for the interpretation of the decline of mortality in later chapters. However it is worth noting that on the assumption that the death rate in 1700 was at or above 30, at least a third of the reduction of the death rate since that time occurred in the pre-registration period.

Table 3.6 also shows the proportion of the decline of mortality in the pre-registration period which was associated with infective conditions: 92 per cent in 1848–54 to 1901; and 73 per cent in 1901 to

1971. On the assumption that there was no decrease of non-infective deaths in the pre-registration period, 86 per cent of the total reduction of the death rate, from the beginning of the eighteenth century to the present day, was attributable to infectious diseases. However, the assumption must be examined carefully.

Non-infective conditions   In the period 1848–54 to 1901, non-infective conditions appear to have contributed 8 per cent to the decline of mortality. Most of this reduction (about four fifths) was associated with two classes of deaths – 'old age' and 'other diseases' – neither of which provides convincing evidence of a true decline. As noted previously, the term 'old age' was used in respect of both infectious and non-infectious deaths, and the fact that in this period there was a considerable increase of deaths certified as bronchitis, pneumonia and influenza and other cardiovascular diseases, suggests that the apparent fall in 'old age' deaths results mainly from a transfer to these categories. The 'other diseases' comprised a large and heterogeneous group of conditions, many of which were unsatisfactorily classified (for example haemorrhage, mortification and insanity). Moreover, the reduction of deaths was mainly in two categories. One consisted of 'asthma and diseases of lungs, etc.' Many of the deaths attributed to these causes were probably associated with respiratory infections, and the apparent decline between 1848–54 and 1901 may have been due mainly to transfers to other categories (such as bronchitis, pneumonia and influenza) as a result of improved certification. The other category of deaths which fell substantially comprised 'debility, atrophy and sudden death, cause unknown'. The first two of these terms are quite unsatisfactory and the reduction of deaths was no doubt due largely to improvements in diagnosis and classification. Although violent deaths are shown separately in the Registrar General's reports, those classified as sudden deaths may have included a considerable number which were caused by violence. About a quarter of these deaths were in the first year of life, so that some may have been due to infanticide. Others, no doubt, were similar to those which would be described today as cot deaths, which means that the cause of death was unknown.

Against this background it seems reasonable to conclude that the Registrar General's statistics provide no convincing evidence of a decline of deaths from non-infective causes between 1848–54 and 1901, and the estimate of 8 per cent (of the total reduction; table 3.6) is probably due mainly to errors in certification of cause of death.

From this conclusion it would seem to follow that the fall of mortality in the pre-registration period was associated almost entirely with infectious diseases. However, there are two non-infective causes of death which may have been important, although this cannot be confirmed from national statistics. I refer to infanticide and starvation.

In his survey of the history of infanticide, Langer concluded that it was practised on a substantial scale in both ancient and modern times.[19] In the eighteenth and nineteenth centuries, 'the poor, hardly able to support the family they already had, evaded responsibility by disposing of further additions.' The same conclusion was reached by many contemporary writers, among them Disraeli who believed that infanticide 'was hardly less prevalent in England than on the banks of the Ganges'. Langer also quotes Ryan who examined the medico-legal aspects of the problem of infanticide and wrote: 'We cannot ignore the fact that the crime of infanticide, as well as that of criminal abortion, is widespread and on the increase.' Although there is no basis for an estimate of the frequency of infanticide, there seems no reason to dissent from Langer's view that it was prevalent at least until the last quarter of the nineteenth century, when it began to be reduced by increasingly stringent regulations, by growing public interest in maternity and child care, and finally by the spread of contraceptive practices.

It is also difficult to assess the frequency of death from starvation, as distinct from death from infectious diseases which resulted from poor nutrition. Although experience in developing countries today suggests that the latter was much more common than the former, it seems probable that in the eighteenth and nineteenth centuries death did occur, at times not infrequently, as a direct result of food deficiency. In the first full year of registration of cause of death, 167 deaths were attributed to starvation. However, an analysis of 63 deaths by Farr showed that the classification was unsatisfactory (they included 12 persons who died from the effects of cold). It is also possible that deaths from starvation were often assigned to other causes.

In spite of the lack of statistical evidence, I believe it is permissible to conclude that death from infanticide was probably common, and death from starvation not uncommon, in the eighteenth and nineteenth centuries. If this is true, mortality from these causes may have declined before registration of cause of death in 1838, and certainly declined after that time. Although this trend cannot be confirmed from national statistics, it is quite possible that these were the only non-infective causes of death associated with a significant reduction of mortality before the twentieth century.

Infective conditions   With the probable exceptions of infanticide and starvation, the decline of mortality before registration, as in the period

---

[19] 'Infanticide: a historical survey', *op. cit.*

from registration to 1900, was due essentially to a reduction of deaths from infectious diseases. As a preliminary to interpretation in subsequent chapters of the reasons for this reduction, it is desirable to come to a conclusion about the nature of the diseases which declined. For the pre-registration period there are no reliable data concerning individual diseases, so again one must draw largely on later experience.

From 1838 the infections which declined were of two types – airborne, and water- and food-borne. Mortality from some of the airborne infections, particularly tuberculosis, fell from the time of registration; however, the fall of mortality from water- and food-borne diseases was delayed until the last decades of the nineteenth century. Although cause of death was registered later in other countries of western Europe than in England and Wales, the evidence for Sweden, France and Ireland is consistent with the conclusion that deaths from water- and food-borne diseases did not begin to decline until about the end of the nineteenth century.[20]

It is probable that there was a substantial reduction of mortality from airborne infections in the pre-registration period. The number of deaths from tuberculosis fell rapidly from 1838, and this disease was associated with nearly half of the total decrease of the death rate during the second half of the nineteenth century. There is little doubt that mortality from tuberculosis was considerable in the seventeenth and eighteenth centuries, and the fact that it was declining at the time of registration suggests that it did so earlier.

The other airborne infection from which deaths must have decreased before 1838 is smallpox. In 1848–54 the death rate from the disease was only 263 (per million), less than a tenth of the rate for respiratory tuberculosis and considerably lower than the rates from whooping cough and measles (table 3.2). We can be less confident about the trend of mortality from other airborne infections in the pre-registration period. Diphtheria was confused with scarlet fever and there is no reliable information about deaths from diseases such as whooping cough, measles, bronchitis, pneumonia and influenza.

Evidence concerning the water- and food-borne diseases is also lacking. Mortality from these infections was not falling in the decades immediately after registration, and did not begin to decline until there were improvements in water supplies and sewage disposal, in England and Wales from the seventh decade and in other countries of western Europe somewhat later.[21] Indeed the appearance of cholera, possibly for the first time, leaves little doubt that in the years after registra-

[20] T. McKeown, R. G. Brown and R. G. Record, 'An interpretation of the modern rise of population in Europe'. *Population Studies*, **26** (1972), p. 345.
[21] *Ibid.*

tion hygienic conditions deteriorated. The rapid movement of populations from country to towns must have led to deterioration of hygiene
and increased exposure to diseases spread by water and food. However, it is quite possible that mortality from water- and food-borne
diseases fell in the pre-registration period, and the grounds for this
conclusion will be discussed in chapter 7.

Finally, I must consider the possible significance of the vector-borne
diseases – plague, typhus and malaria – spread by rats, lice and
mosquitoes respectively. These diseases were relatively unimportant
after registration: plague almost disappeared from the British Isles
after 1679, and although cases were introduced occasionally through
seaports, no extension of the disease occurred; typhus was not separated
from typhoid before 1869 and few deaths were attributed to it after
that time; and although there may have been some indigenous cases
of malaria, most of the deaths have resulted from infections acquired
overseas.

If judged by the attention paid to it by historians, plague was
much the most important of the vector-borne diseases in relation to
the decline of mortality and growth of population before registration.
Since the disease virtually disappeared after 1679, it cannot have been
associated with the decrease of deaths in the next two centuries. But
it has been suggested that plague may nevertheless have been significant, on the grounds that it provided a check on population
growth in earlier centuries, a check which was removed by the failure
of the disease to reappear.

The credibility of this hypothesis turns on several issues, including
particularly the importance of plague as a cause of death before the
eighteenth century. By simple arithmetic it can be shown that a high
death rate from an infrequent epidemic infection has much less effect
on the general level of mortality and rate of population growth than
the constant high death rate from endemic infections which killed the
majority of all newborn children within ten years of birth. Moreover, in his *History of Bubonic Plague* Shrewsbury rejected some of the
estimates of plague mortality made by historians.[22] Armed with a
knowledge of the biology of the bacterium and the natural history of
the disease, he concluded *inter alia*: that no pestilence (in the British
Isles) before the fourteenth century can be identified as plague; that it
was biologically impossible for the whole or even a major part of
England to have been ravaged by 'the Great Pestilence' of 1348–50
and that the latter was confined to the southern and eastern counties;
that this epidemic affected only the smaller part of the population

[22] J. F. D. Shrewsbury, *A history of bubonic plague in the British Isles.* Cambridge University Press
(Cambridge, 1970), pp. 13, 24, 28, 36, 123, 127, 478, 486/7.

of England, and that statements that it destroyed three quarters or even one half of the nation are flights of fancy boosted by the age old terror that the name plague still exerts; that in the comparatively densely populated region of East Anglia and in the larger towns that were affected by it, 'the Great Pestilence' may possibly have destroyed as much as one third of the population, but for the country as a whole the death rate did not exceed one twentieth. Shrewsbury also concluded that the later pestilences in the second half of the fourteenth century were not plague, and that the disease caused only one or two local epidemics and few deaths in the fifteenth century.

Nevertheless Shrewsbury agreed that there were numerous outbreaks of bubonic plague throughout the sixteenth and seventeenth centuries and that some of them resulted in heavy mortality. Even so, his estimates of the death rates attributable to the disease are lower than many others. For example, he suggested that the rates in London in the most severe epidemics were: 1563, 25 per cent; 1593, 12 per cent; 1603, 19 per cent; 1625, 16 per cent; 1665, 17 per cent. In plague years a substantial proportion of the deaths was due to other causes, which over any considerable area and period of time were predominent in determining the general level of mortality. On these grounds Shrewsbury rejected the critical influence suggested for plague on population growth: 'One fallacy about the effect of bubonic plague upon London in particular and England in general that has been given considerable publicity is that the mortality caused by it was responsible for the slow growth of the English population in the seventeenth century.' But even if plague had a greater part in limiting the growth of population in the sixteenth and seventeenth centuries than Shrewsbury was prepared to assign to it, if we accept his conclusions about experience of the disease in the fourteenth and fifteenth centuries, it cannot be regarded as the critical influence whose withdrawal was largely responsible for the rise of population after 1700.

There has been no comparable work on the history of the other vector-borne diseases once prevalent in England. Typhus was not differentiated from bubonic plague until about the middle of the nineteenth century and according to Shrewsbury was responsible for many of the deaths attributed to that disease. As already mentioned, typhus was confused with typhoid in national statistics in the years after registration. Malaria also could not be identified reliably from many other fevers before the late nineteenth century, and in the early Registrar General's reports it does not appear as such and was presumably included under terms such as intermittent fever. In view of the lack of evidence one can attempt only a personal appraisal. I conclude no more than that there were epidemics of typhus, particularly affecting the poor, at intervals during the pre-registration period, and that mortality declined until the disease virtually disappeared in the late nineteenth century; that malaria was never an important cause of death in Britain (where climatic conditions are not really suited to the malaria parasite) and the disease was not associated significantly with the reduction of mortality in the pre-registration period.

In this interpretation, vector-borne diseases are assigned a much less significant place in the history of mortality and population growth in England, and indeed in most of Europe, than the one they occupy in developing countries today. The reason is clear. Most developing countries are in or near the tropics, where climatic conditions are ideal for many parasites and animal vectors – particularly flies, mosquitoes and snails – with the result that diseases such as dysentery, malaria, yellow fever and bilharzia are endemic over large areas. But in western Europe, even in past centuries conditions were far from ideal for the diseases spread by animal vectors. For example, a temperature of not less than 20°C is required before the sexual cycle of plasmodium falciparum (the cause of malignant subtertian malaria) can be completed in the mosquito, and a temperature of 15° is needed for other species. For this reason it is unlikely that malaria was ever common in Britain. In another sense than they intended, there is truth in the Webbs' observation that England (like most of Europe) has the worst weather and the best climate in the world.

I must now bring together these rather fragmentary conclusions concerning the diseases associated with the decline of mortality since the beginning of the eighteenth century. On the assumption that the death rate in 1700 was about 30, the proportion of the fall of mortality which occurred in three periods was: 1700 to 1848–54 (the pre-registration period), 33 per cent; 1848–54 to 1901, 20 per cent; 1901 to 1971, 47 per cent. The decline of the death rate was associated predominantly with infectious diseases. It is probable that there was a reduction of deaths from infanticide and starvation in the eighteenth and nineteenth centuries, but with these exceptions there is no convincing evidence of a decrease of deaths from non-infective conditions before 1900. From then until 1971 the latter were associated with approximately a quarter of the decline of mortality.

Of the fall of mortality in the post-registration period, 40 per cent was due to airborne diseases, 21 per cent to water- and food-borne diseases, 13 per cent to other infections and the remainder (26 per cent) to non-infective conditions; the contribution of individual diseases, or groups of diseases, in each of these classes is shown in tables 3.2, 3.3, 3.4 and 3.5 respectively. Many of the conditions included under other infections were unsatisfactorily classified and it is probable that most of them were airborne.

With the exceptions of infanticide and starvation, the reduction of mortality in the pre-registration period was also associated with the infections. Although information about individual diseases is lacking, there is little doubt that mortality from at least two major airborne infections – tuberculosis and smallpox – had fallen before 1838. There is reason to believe that there was also a significant decrease of deaths from water- and food-borne diseases (discussed in chapter 7). Of the vector-borne diseases, plague had virtually disappeared before the beginning of the eighteenth century, and it is unlikely that malaria was ever an important cause of death in the British Isles; however, the decline of typhus undoubtedly contributed to the reduction of mortality in the pre-registration period.

To summarize: the decline of mortality since the end of the seventeenth century was due predominantly to a reduction of deaths associated with infectious diseases. The diseases chiefly concerned were airborne infections, probably throughout the whole period, and water- and food-borne diseases in the eighteenth century and again from the late nineteenth. The contribution of the vector-borne diseases – mainly typhus – to the decline was almost restricted to the pre-registration period and was relatively small. Among non-infective conditions, there was a reduction of deaths from infanticide and starvation in the eighteenth and nineteenth centuries and from a number of other causes of death during the twentieth.

The four chapters which follow are concerned with interpretation of the decline of mortality from infectious diseases. The significance of the trend of deaths from non-infective conditions, including infanticide and starvation, will be considered in chapter 8.

4
Infective organisms and human hosts

The conclusion that the modern rise of population was due essentially to a decrease of mortality, which resulted from a reduction of deaths caused by infectious diseases, brings us to a central issue in the demography of the past three centuries, namely the reasons for the decline of the infections. In broad terms the problem may be stated as follows. It is probable that the predominance of infectious diseases dates from the first agricultural revolution when men began to aggregate in populations of considerable size. Why then did the infections decline from about the time of the Industrial Revolution which led to the aggregation of still larger and more densely packed populations? The answer to this paradox must be sought in the character of micro-organisms, the conditions under which they spread and the response of the human host, inherited or acquired.

However, for an understanding of the infections it is unsatisfactory to consider separately an organism and its host. They are living things which interact and adapt to each other by natural selection. The virulence of an organism is not, therefore, a distinct character like its size or shape; it is an expression of an interaction between a particular organism and a particular host. For example, a measles virus whose effects on children in a developed country are relatively benign, may have devastating effects when encountered by a population for the first time, as occurred in the nineteenth century in Fiji and the Faeroes. When assessing the major influences on the infections it will therefore be necessary to distinguish clearly between the following.

(a) The interaction between organism and host. When exposed to micro-organisms over a period of time, the hosts gain through natural selection an intrinsic resistance which is genetically determined. In addition to this intrinsic resistance immunity may also be acquired, by transmission from the mother or in response to a postnatal infection. These types of immunity, inherited and acquired, are not due to either medical intervention or, as a rule, to identifiable environmental influences.

(b) Immunization and therapy. Immunity to infection may also result from successful immunization, and the outcome of an established infection may be influenced by therapy.

(c) Modes of spread. The modes of spread are very different for different micro-organisms, and the feasibility of controlling a communicable disease by preventing contact with the organism is determined largely by the way it is transmitted. In a developed country it is relatively easy to prevent the spread of cholera by purification of water; it is more difficult to control salmonella infection by supervision of food handling; and at present it is impossible to eliminate an airborne infection such as the common cold by preventing exposure to the virus.

(d) The nutrition of the host. The results of an encounter with a micro-organism are influenced not only by the inherited or acquired immunity of the host, but also by his general state of health determined particularly, it will be suggested, by nutrition.

This classification provides a basis for an analysis of reasons for the decline of the infectious diseases. It is against the background of an understanding of the interaction between organism and host that we must consider the possibility that the decline was due substantially to a change in the character of infectious diseases, essentially independent of both medical intervention and identifiable environmental (including nutritional) improvements. It is in relation to immunization and therapy that we must assess the contribution of specific medical measures. A judgement on the significance of reduction of exposure to infection must rest on an understanding of the modes of spread of micro-organisms. And an estimate of the importance of an increase in food supplies depends upon appraisal of the association between malnutrition and infection. The contribution of these influences to the decline of mortality from infectious diseases will be discussed in this and the three chapters which follow.

INTERACTION BETWEEN ORGANISM AND HOST

With due regard for some uncertainties concerning the evolution of micro-organisms, there is no doubt that they have evolved together with and, in a sense, in balance with their hosts. By natural selection the hosts acquire resistance to organisms which cause disease, by their ability to produce an immune response and by the more general type of intrinsic resistance which makes an individual immune to a particular organism. It is this last type of immunity which explains why shigella dysentery is confined to primates and Johne's disease to ruminants; why most children exposed to poliomyelitis virus do not suffer from the disease;

and why tuberculosis is a natural infection of man, cattle, pigs and fowls but is relatively uncommon in sheep, goats, horses and dogs. By natural selection micro-organisms also adapt, and the relationship can be said to be in balance in the sense that there are reciprocal changes in organism and host. The clinical outcome in a particular infection depends on the interplay of these reactions of parasite and host, and varies from complete subjugation of the host to destruction of the micro-organism, including near stalemate in chronic infections.[1] Andrewes cites rabbit myxomatosis as an example of balanced evolution of host and parasite:[2]

Infection is transmitted mechanically by a biting insect, whether mosquito in Australia or flea in Britain. Virus is not adequately picked up from the blood, but only from where it is most abundantly present, in the myxomatous lumps in the skin. Unless these appear and are reasonably rich in virus, spread will not occur. In Australia the originally introduced virus killed more than 99 per cent of the rabbits it infected. After a very few years, however, less virulent strains appeared and soon predominated over the virulent ones. What happened is fairly clear. A less vicious virus permitted the infected rabbit to live longer: it was thus available for a longer time as a source of virus for biting mosquitoes, and was therefore spread more widely than the original virus. The tendency was therefore towards a progressive attenuation of virus – yet that could not go too far: if the virus was too mild there would be no virus-rich lumps for infecting more insects. Rather unexpectedly, the rabbits themselves, through selection of naturally more resistant animals, began very quickly to acquire a genetic resistance to the virus so that only 60–70 per cent were being killed – nothing to worry about for a rabbit which really knows how to breed fast. Now, however, in the more resistant rabbits the attenuated strains which were doing so nicely at one time were not producing adequately rich lumps, so the evolutionary changes went into reverse, greater virulence being required. In short the virulence of the virus and the resistance of the host seem able to vary and adjust themselves, the product of their activity being a particular disease picture; this alone remains fairly stable at a level which permits virus to spread effectively without killing too many rabbits.

This account of balanced evolution illustrates that the relation between a micro-organism and its host is not fixed but is constantly

[1] H. Smith, 'Host factors influencing microbial proliferation *in vivo*'. In *Resistance to Infectious Disease*, edited by R. H. Dunlop and H. W. Moon, Saskatoon Modern Press (1970), p. 144.
[2] C. Andrewes, 'Viruses and evolution'. The Huxley Lecture, 1965–6, University of Birmingham (1966).

changing, as a result of the interaction between nature and nurture in both host and parasite. It should also be noted that the stability of the relationship is not the same for different organisms. It is particularly volatile in the case of the streptococcus, and this explains the several cycles of severity and benignity which have been observed in the history of scarlet fever. However, there are other organisms for which the relationship is more stable; for example, there appear to have been no significant changes in the virulence of the tubercle bacillus during the period in which it has been assessed in the laboratory. In such cases the relation between organism and host is of course only relatively more constant, and over any considerable period it also changes.

It is important to consider at this point the circumstances under which contact with a micro-organism causes disease. In general it is not to the advantage of micro-organisms to kill their hosts, and Andrewes notes that many, probably most virus infections are latent and some may be beneficial. However, there are organisms whose spread and survival depend on the sickness of their hosts: the common cold is spread by sneezing; cholera by diarrhoea; respiratory tuberculosis by coughing; and rabies by the biting of dogs. While such examples are common among organisms which cause sickness and death, they are uncommon among micro-organisms as a whole.

Disease of the host may also result when an organism is encountered by a population for the first time or after an interval of several generations, and this presumably occurs with the so-called epidemic communicable diseases such as plague, typhus or influenza. In the case of viruses Andrewes noted that when an infection is introduced to a strange host, for example as a result of an insect bite, one of three things may happen.[2] The virus may fail to multiply and this, probably the commonest outcome, passes unnoticed. Or the virus may multiply and kill the host without being transmitted to another, in which case the infection ends at this point; this is also very common in experience of viruses. The third possibility is that after a period of adaptation, accompanied initially by morbidity and even death of some hosts and parasites, the virus and host settle to a relation of mutual tolerance normally not associated with disease. In the light of this interpretation it is clearly unreasonable to think of the microbe as the aggressor and the host as the passive and innocent victim, a point which would have appealed to Montaigne who wrote: 'When I play with my cat, who knows but that she regards me more as a plaything than I do her.'

Although Andrewes's account of the results of contact between host and parasite is based on viruses, there is no reason to think that the mechanism is essentially different in the case of other micro-organisms. In the present context the important conclusions are that most contacts between organisms and their potential hosts end blindly and, when they do not, after a period of adaptation the infections often do not lead to disease. That is to say that the picture of morbidity and death associated with communicable disease. is misleading, since it represents only a small and selected part of the total experience with micro-organisms.

A detailed description of the mechanisms of immunity would be out of place in the present discussion, but as a background to the examination of reasons for the decline of the infections it will be desirable to consider briefly the different ways in which the resistance of a host may be increased. It is particularly important to distinguish between (a) immunity which is inherited or acquired naturally, either from the mother or through infection by micro-organisms, (b) immunity induced artificially by immunization or serum transfer and (c) resistance which is determined by the host's general health, influenced particularly by nutrition. Here we are concerned only with the first of these mechanisms; the second and third are considered in chapters 5 and 7 respectively.

The types of immunity referred to under (a) may, with reservations, be said to be natural, in the sense that they are determined genetically or result from experience of disease, rather than from direct human intervention. Nevertheless it should be recognized that neither of these mechanisms is wholly independent of the environment. For example, poor nutrition in a population may lead to heavy mortality from tuberculosis; this mortality in one generation influences, through natural selection, the genetically determined resistance to the disease in the next. Also, improved hygiene may reduce the number of people who encounter typhoid, and so limit the proportion who acquire immunity by having been infected. But with these reservations, the types of resistance which occur naturally are distinguishable from those which can be brought about directly by human intervention ((b) and (c) above). They are of three kinds.

Probably the most important type of immunity is that which makes a species resistant to a micro-organism or its toxins. This resistance may be absolute, in the sense that the species shows no evidence of contact with a micro-organism; or it may be relative, as is usually the case with the individual or racial differences which occur within a species. In general the differences in resistance within a species are less marked than those between species; and together the two types of inherited resistance are much more important than those which are acquired. It is because of the protection conferred by this form of immunity that most micro-organisms are prevented from establishing themselves as parasites. With few exceptions, the characteristics of the host which determine this innate immunity are unknown.

Apart from medical intervention, immunity may be acquired by transmission of antibodies from the mother to the foetus or newborn infant. This mechanism protects the child in the early months of life against the infections to which the mother has been exposed.

Resistance may also be acquired naturally as a result of infection by a micro-organism, but the degree of protection varies widely. Repeated attacks are very rare in the case of measles, smallpox and diphtheria; they are relatively common after influenza, pneumonia or the common cold.

This short appraisal of the interaction between organism and host leads to some conclusions which are important for the examination of reasons for the decline of the infections: that parasites and hosts have evolved in balance and the relation between them is constantly changing; that it is only in special circumstances that micro-organisms cause disease; and that animals, including man, are protected from micro-organisms and their toxins by inherited and, to a lesser extent, acquired immunity. These conclusions have a considerable bearing on speculation concerning the disappearance of plague and on the larger question whether the decline of the infections can be attributed substantially to a change in the character of infectious diseases.

INFECTIOUS DISEASES OF EARLY MAN

Before discussing the possibility that a change in the character of the infections contributed substantially to the decline of mortality since the eighteenth century, it will be desirable to consider briefly early man's experience of infectious disease. It is particularly important to come to a conclusion about the significance of the infections during man's evolution, and to assess the changes in the diseases which resulted from the aggregation of populations after the first agricultural revolution.

During most of his existence man has been a comparatively rare animal living in small groups of no more than a few hundred persons. Such conditions do not permit the transmission and survival of many micro-organisms, and some years ago Burnet suggested that infectious diseases as we now know them did not exist:[3]

> It is generally considered that in the early stages of human evolution primitive man and his subhuman progenitors existed in small wandering groups of at most a few families, and that these groups only rarely came into contact one with the other. Under such circumstances it would be virtually impossible for a pathogen to evolve as a specifically human parasite unless, as is the case with herpes simplex, the period over which a person remained capable of transferring infection was of the order of a generation . . .

[3] F. M. Burnet, *Virus as Organism*. Harvard University Press (Cambridge, 1946), pp. 30–31.

To return to the question of the specifically human virus disease: we have given reasons for believing that in the early phase of human existence, from the beginning of the pleistocene up to about 10,000 years ago, infectious disease due to micro-organisms specifically adapted to the human species was almost nonexistent. The herpes virus could have persisted with very much its present type of activity, but the viruses producing brief infection with subsequent immunity – measles, mumps, and the like – could obviously not have survived in anything like their present form.

However, although knowledge of infections in the wild is still very incomplete, it is now clear that some human parasites had precursors in other primates. This subject has been discussed extensively by Cockburn, who cites many examples of precursors including intestinal protozoa, worms, lice, malaria parasites, the scabies mite, herpes virus, infective hepatitis virus and possibly syphilis and other treponematoses.[4]

There is no reason to doubt that early man was exposed to the zoonoses, that is to infections of other animals transmitted to man by ticks, mites, mosquitoes and other biting arthropods. Cockburn suggests that anthrax, botulism and possibly leprosy occurred in this way. Andrewes has drawn attention to the central place occupied by arthropods, particularly insects, in the history of viruses.[2] It is not surprising that arthropods, which probably comprise the largest number of the earth's inhabitants other than micro-organisms, should have provided suitable conditions for the propagation and transmission of viruses.

The first agricultural revolution was accompanied by changes which must have affected profoundly man's experience of infectious disease; these included, for example, loss of mobility, increase in food supplies, domestication of animals and conditions of life which attracted intruders such as the rat, mouse, sparrow, tick, flea and mosquito. But perhaps the most significant influence was the increase both in total population size and in the size of local groups in close personal contact. Many infections require minimal host populations if they are to be maintained, and it was only after the first agricultural revolution that human populations reached the size needed for the perpetuation of many organisms which have no animal host. They include some of the prominent infections of today – mumps, measles, chicken pox, rubella and smallpox. The importance of population size is illustrated by experience of measles. The disease was introduced to the Faeroes in 1846 with serious results, but the population (7000) was too small to maintain the infection. On the basis of American experience Cockburn has suggested that a population of about 1,000,000 is near the threshold

[4] T. A. Cockburn, 'Infectious diseases in ancient populations'. *Current Anthropology*, **12** (1971).

required to support measles as an endemic infection. Clearly populations of this size have existed only during the past few thousand years.

It is difficult to confirm these conclusions by observations of people who have retained a primitive way of life to the present day, most of whom have been in contact with the external world. However, it is interesting that a hunting people of Tanganyika showed evidence only of infections which could survive in a small population always on the move, until others such as measles, rubella and chicken pox were introduced by contact with larger populations.[5]

In summary, with due regard for the lack of direct evidence, it seems probable that early man suffered from some infectious diseases which are found in other primates, and from others contracted from animal vectors, usually arthropods. Living in small groups he is unlikely to have experienced many of the infections which are prominent today, particularly those which are airborne (measles, mumps, smallpox, tuberculosis, influenza, diphtheria and the common cold). The rise of airborne diseases, including notably the respiratory infections, probably dates from the time when human populations first aggregated in groups of substantial size.

This interpretation explains why the infectious diseases became predominant as causes of death from the time of the first agricultural revolution. In the following chapters I shall suggest why they declined from about the time of the second.

CHANGES IN THE INFECTIOUS DISEASES SINCE THE EIGHTEENTH CENTURY

I must now consider the question: Was the decline of the infections during the past few centuries due to any considerable extent to a change in the character of the diseases, that is, to a modification of the relation between micro-organisms and their hosts of the kind discussed in the opening pages of this chapter? Such a modification is not independent of the environment; indeed it is determined largely by an ecological relationship to the environment. It is however a change such as must have occurred continuously during man's history, and was essentially independent both of medical intervention by immunization or therapy, and of identifiable environmental measures such as better hygiene and improved nutrition.

Some biologists have thought that a change in the character of infectious diseases was important, and one or two have concluded that it was the main reason for the decline of mortality and improvement

---

[5] D. B. Jelliffe, J. Woodburn, F. J. Bennett and E. F. P. Jelliffe, 'The children of the Hadza hunters'. *Tropical Paediatrics*, **60**, p. 907.

in health. An extreme statement of this viewpoint was contained in Magill's presidential address to the American Association of Immuno-logists in 1954.[6] In it he questioned the efficacy of therapy and suggested: 'It would seem to be a more logical conclusion that during recent years, quite regardless of our therapeutic efforts, a state of relative equilibrium has established itself between the microbes and the "ever-varying state of the immunological constitution of the herd" – a relative equilibrium which will continue, perhaps, just as long as it is not disturbed, unduly, by biological events.' According to this interpretation, the trend of mortality from infectious diseases has been essentially independent of both medical measures and the vast economic and social developments of the past three centuries.

The grounds on which it was possible to reach so radical a viewpoint are important and have been largely overlooked or, according to Magill, ignored. He based his conclusions on the ineffectiveness and dangers of vaccination against rabies, the decline of tuberculosis long before effec-tive treatment, the behaviour of diphtheria in the nineteenth century (it increased in prevalence and malignancy in the middle of the century and declined before the introduction of antitoxin), and the rapid reduc-tion of pneumonia death rates in New York State before the 'miracle' drugs were known, followed by an arrest of the decline from about the time when antibiotics were introduced. Moreover these examples of the ineffectiveness of medical measures could be extended. For example, the cholera vaccine required until recently by international regulations, is almost useless; the reduction of mortality from diphtheria in the 1940s did not everywhere coincide with the introduction of immuniza-tion; and scarlet fever is an example of a disease whose variable history appears to have been independent of medical and other identifiable influences.

Nevertheless, although there is no doubt that specific medical mea-sures have had little effect on the behaviour of many infections, the question concerning the significance of changes in the character of the infectious diseases is too complex and too important to be dismissed without careful examination. But before examining these issues in more detail I should clarify the implications of the suggestion that the decline of mortality from the infections was due substantially to a favourable change in the 'ever-varying state of the immunological constitution of the herd'.

The immunological constitution of a generation is influenced largely by the mortality experience of those which precede it. This was par-ticularly true in past centuries, when the majority of liveborn individuals

[6] T. P. Magill, 'The immunologist and the evil spirits'. *Journal of Immunology*, **74** (1955), p. 1.

died from infectious disease without reproducing. Under such conditions there was rigorous natural selection in respect of immunity to infection. The proposal that the decline of mortality resulted from improvement in the immunological constitution of the population therefore implies that there was heavy mortality at an earlier period which led to the birth of individuals who were genetically less susceptible. According to this interpretation, the substantial and prolonged decline of infectious deaths was brought about, not by improvements which have occurred since the eighteenth century, but by an earlier deterioration of conditions which led to the high mortality which must have preceded it. I shall now consider the implications of this conclusion in relation to airborne, water- and food-borne and vector-borne diseases.

Airborne diseases
There are two reasons for beginning with the airborne diseases, first because they contributed most to the decline of mortality since the eighteenth century (table 3.1) and second, because they appear to have become predominant at the time of the first agricultural revolution. Is it possible that their predominance since then was due to a change in the character of the diseases, and that this change has been reversed since the eighteenth century?

There is no reason to doubt that the airborne infections became important because domestication of plants and animals led to the aggregation of populations of the size required for their propagation and survival. And although conditions of life have varied greatly since that time, population size has remained large enough in many places for the diseases to continue as major causes of sickness and death. The relative importance of different airborne diseases has of course varied between populations and at different periods. I must now enquire whether the decline of these infections from about the time of the Industrial Revolution, in spite of the aggregation of still larger populations, was due to a change in their character, by which is meant a reduction of the virulence of the micro-organisms or an increase of the resistance, mainly genetically determined, of their hosts. These issues will be considered by reference to four airborne diseases – scarlet fever, influenza, tuberculosis and measles.

Scarlet fever is the outstanding example of an infection in which the relation between host and parasite is unstable, and the decline of mortality since the mid nineteenth century can be attributed confidently to a change in the character of the disease. This is the conclusion reached by those who have considered the history of scarlet fever, since it was first described by Sydenham in 1676, as a mild disease. It has exhibited at least four cycles of severity and remission. It was very serious in the late eighteenth century, and again in the mid nineteenth century, when it was at its worst about 1863. Mortality fell rapidly in the next forty years, but it was still an important cause of death at the beginning of the present century. Since then it has declined, and is today a relatively minor illness. Against the background of this history we cannot be confident that it will always remain so.

Influenza is another disease whose severity has fluctuated. It is hardly necessary to emphasize its past, and almost certainly continuing, importance. It is the only epidemic infectious disease which, in techno-logically advanced countries, presents today a threat comparable to that experienced in earlier centuries from diseases such as plague and typhus. Its occurrence is quite unpredictable, and its severity varies from epidemic to epidemic, apparently quite independently of medical measures or identifiable environmental influences. This variation is determined largely by variation in the types of influenza virus.

In tuberculosis also it has been suggested that man's relation to the organism has varied, and indeed that the fall of mortality since cause of death was first registered in 1838 can be interpreted as the end of an epidemic wave. There is no evidence that the virulence of the organism has changed significantly; the disease continues to have devastating effects on populations not previously exposed to it; and the virulence of the bacillus appears not to have diminished during the period when it has been possible to assess it in the laboratory. The question is therefore whether the decline of mortality was due substantially to an increase in man's genetically determined resistance to the disease.

Both evidence from twins and the response of populations not pre-viously exposed leave no doubt that susceptibility to tuberculosis is in a considerable degree genetically determined. But it does not follow that the decline of mortality was due to genetic selection. The effects of selection are maximum after first exposure, and it is not easy to see how it could account for a dramatic change in a population which had been exposed to the disease for several centuries. Theoretically, however, there are two ways in which selection might have contributed.

One way is by the break-up of isolates. This possibility was discussed by Dahlberg: 'If susceptibility to tuberculosis is conditioned by reces-sive genes, the break-up of isolates should cause the disease to become more infrequent, since the frequency of allelic genes in duplicate doses thereby decreases. Another way of expressing the same thing is to say that the break-up of isolates decreases the frequency of consanguineous marriages, and thereby also the frequency of homozygotes. Such a mechanism must clearly have played some part, particularly in countries with a more highly developed and extensive industry where cities have grown at the expense of the rural populations.'[7]

[7] G. Dahlberg, 'Mortality from tuberculosis in some countries'. *British Journal of Social Medicine*, **3** (1955), p. 220.

But while the break-up of isolates may have contributed to the reduction of mortality from rare conditions, it is very unlikely to have had much effect on a disease as common as tuberculosis. Indeed, if dispersal of rural populations was significant, it is a second possibility that must be considered more seriously – the effect of selection on rural populations not previously exposed.

Is it likely that although tuberculosis was common in Britain during the seventeenth and eighteenth centuries, the disease was mainly restricted to towns? If so, a large part of the rural population might not have been exposed, so that the decline of mortality could reflect largely the effects of selection on those meeting the disease for the first time. This explanation rests on three assumptions.

1 That before the Industrial Revolution a substantial proportion of the rural population had not encountered tuberculosis.

2. That improved communications and the movement into towns resulted in first exposure and death of many susceptible individuals. However, the movement to towns was not at the right time or – initially – of sufficient magnitude to be consistent with this explanation. At least from the beginning of registration of cause of death, the decline of mortality from tuberculosis was very rapid; it fell by a quarter in the fifth decade of the nineteenth century. To have contributed largely to this change, selection would have had to operate in respect of almost the whole population at least thirty years earlier. Yet by 1801, only 17 per cent (by 1831, 25 per cent) of the population of England and Wales were living in towns with 20,000 or more people.

3 That mortality from the disease increased sharply in the late eighteenth and early nineteenth centuries. Again the statistical evidence is quite inadequate. But to have had a selective effect of the requisite dimensions, the rise in mortality would have to have been very great indeed. Moreover its subsequent decline would be only in respect of the newly exposed population and would certainly not be expected to continue to or below the level of the early eighteenth century (the level determined by that part of the population which had been exposed to the disease for centuries).

I conclude that genetic selection is unlikely to have contributed substantially to the decline of mortality from tuberculosis in Britain since 1838. Indeed it is possible that in recent years the resistance of populations of advanced countries has diminished, since selection in respect of it is much less rigorous than formerly, and there are many people who have never acquired resistance postnatally by exposure to the disease.

In the same context, experience of measles is also instructive. Childhood mortality from the disease was relatively high during the nineteenth and early twentieth centuries, but declined rapidly from about the time of the First World War. Nevertheless as noted previously (p. 59), measles remains an important infectious disease.

Although no completely satisfactory interpretation has been given, or perhaps can be expected, for the enormous reduction in mortality from measles which occurred in, roughly, the past fifty years, some points are not in doubt. One is that where the disease kills large numbers of children, resistance to it is increased by natural selection. This explains the difference in response to the same virus in a western population previously exposed, and in a developed country meeting the disease for the first time. Also, while the disease was known for many centuries, it is probable that the aggregation of populations which occurred in the nineteenth century created optimum conditions for the survival and spread of the virus. It is therefore possible that industrialization led to increased mortality from measles, and that the subsequent decline owed something to increased resistance to the disease in later generations, genetically determined and brought about by natural selection. In measles, unlike tuberculosis, the beginning of the fall of mortality was late enough to be consistent with this conclusion. However, it will be suggested later (chapter 7) that there are grounds for believing that this was not the only, or probably the most important, influence on the trend of mortality from the disease.

On the basis of experience of these four diseases it is possible to assess the likelihood that the reduction of deaths from airborne diseases was due substantially to a change in their character. Scarlet fever and influenza are examples of endemic and epidemic infections respectively, whose severity has fluctuated at relatively short intervals, apparently unaffected by medical measures or identifiable environmental influences. The fluctuations in mortality may therefore be attributed to variation in the character of the diseases, that is to a change in the relationship between the micro-organisms and their human hosts. But the cycles of these changes have been of relatively short duration, and while they may have affected the trend of mortality considerably over short periods (influenza over a few years, scarlet fever over many decades), over longer periods the increases and decreases of deaths are of the same order and have had little effect on the long term trend. This conclusion must be accepted for infectious diseases in general before the eighteenth century; that is to say the fluctuation in mortality associated with changes in the character of the diseases must have roughly cancelled out, to account for the continued high level of the death rate.

In tuberculosis and measles the issues are different. There is no evidence that these diseases have fluctuated in severity since the eighteenth century and, although mortality from both has declined, it has done so over different periods. Death rates from tuberculosis have fallen rapidly and continuously since they were first registered in 1838. For the reduction to have been caused by a change in the character of the disease brought about by natural selection, there would need to have been a large increase in mortality from tuberculosis in the eighteenth century. In measles, however, the decrease of deaths began in the second decade of the twentieth century, and the possibility cannot be excluded that it resulted in part from earlier high mortality which followed the increase in population size in the industrial towns. It is also relevant that in tuberculosis and measles, unlike scarlet fever and influenza, it is possible to identify other influences which contributed largely to the decline of mortality.

Against this background I conclude that while there is no airborne infection – indeed there is no infection – of which one can say confidently that there has been no change in the relation between the micro-organism and host since the eighteenth century, there are some such as tuberculosis and, probably, measles in which this is very unlikely to be the main reason for the decrease of deaths. But the objection to this as the major influence on all airborne infections is of a more general kind. To believe that the reduction of deaths from these diseases was due essentially to a change in their character, we should have to accept either (a) that fortuitously, over the whole range of airborne diseases, there was a change of the kind which appears to have occurred in scarlet fever, independent of medical or other identifiable influences, or (b) that certain deleterious influences – presumably associated with industrialization – led to high mortality in the eighteenth century, which, through natural selection, resulted in the survival of more resistant populations. In the light of the extent and duration of the fall of mortality the first explanation is incredible. And since there is no evidence that mortality increased greatly in the eighteenth century the second explanation is also untenable.

Water- and food-borne diseases

Some of the issues related to the character of water- and food-borne diseases are analogous to those discussed above in respect of airborne infections. The relation of the organisms to their hosts is variable, so that over any considerable period there are changes in the character of the diseases which appear to be independent of identifiable influences. It is also true that where there is high mortality from a disease such as typhoid, natural selection results in the birth of more resistant populations. Is it likely that this was a significant influence on the rapid fall of deaths from these diseases which began in the late nineteenth century?

Hygienic conditions deteriorated in the first half of the nineteenth century, as a result of rapid growth of towns with uncontrolled domestic and industrial conditions. It is therefore by no means unlikely that mortality from water- and food-borne diseases increased for a time, and that later populations were to some extent selected for their resistance to the organisms. But there are two reasons for believing that this was not a major influence on the decline of mortality. In the first place there is no evidence of a large increase of mortality from the diseases, of the kind needed to account substantially for the later decrease. And secondly, another and more convincing explanation is available, namely, the improvements in hygiene which will be discussed in chapter 6. This illustrates the advantage of examining water- and food-borne infections separately from those that are airborne. A change in the character of airborne diseases has to be considered with regard for the fact that exposure to the organisms cannot be prevented. But in the case of water- and food-borne diseases, separation from the source of infection was the critical measure in their control. While, therefore, we cannot exclude the possibility that typhoid and dysentery at the end of the nineteenth century differed somewhat from the same diseases in the early industrial towns, it is unlikely that any difference was a major reason for the rapid reduction of mortality from the intestinal infections which followed improvements in water supply and sewage disposal.

Vector-borne diseases

As already noted, typhus is the vector-borne disease whose decline may have contributed significantly to the fall of mortality in Britain, mainly in the eighteenth and early nineteenth centuries. As in the case of other epidemic infections, knowledge of the multiple factors which determined its disappearance and reappearance is still incomplete. But we cannot rule out the possibility that among them was a change in the character of the disease, apparently unrelated to medical measures or identifiable environmental influences. However, even if the decrease of deaths from typhus could be accounted for largely in this way, the contribution of the vector-borne diseases to the decline of mortality as a whole would have been small.

Since bubonic plague has not been seen in the British Isles since the seventeenth century, it would seem unnecessary to consider it in an interpretation of the decline of mortality from the eighteenth. However, it has been suggested that the disappearance of plague was important in the demographic history of Britain, and that its failure to return may explain the beginning of the modern rise of population.

There are several reasons for questioning this conclusion. As mentioned in the preceding chapter, Shrewsbury doubted the importance assigned to plague by some historians. He also outlined, in characteristically forthright terms, the reasons for its disappearance: 'Bubonic plague disappeared from London and from England because the maritime importation of Pasteurella pestis in plague-infected ship rats from European and Levantine ports ceased. Plague disappeared from western and central Europe also during the latter half of this century for the same reason, to wit, the development of the all-sea trade between Europe and India, which abolished the caravan route for merchandise from the East across Asia Minor and with it the "rodent pipe-line" for the transit of P. pestis from its Indian homeland to the ports of the Levant.'[8] This interpretation attributes the disappearance of plague, not to a change in the character of the disease, but to elimination of the risk of exposure.

This is a suitable point at which to consider more closely the suggestion that the disappearance of plague had an important bearing on subsequent demographic history.[9] Assuming that the disappearance of the disease was due to the interruption of land trade routes, as suggested by Shrewsbury, if this had not occurred it is possible that plague would have returned to western Europe in the eighteenth century. Had it done so mortality would have been somewhat higher and the rate of population growth correspondingly lower. But if we accept Shrewsbury's estimates of plague mortality in previous centuries, these effects would not have been large.

In relation to the modern rise of population as a whole, the significance of a return of plague would have been even more restricted. With the possible exception of tuberculosis, no single disease was critical for the decline of mortality; the vector-borne diseases were far less important in western Europe than those which were air-, water- and food-borne; and the occasional epidemic infections contributed much less to the general level of mortality than the endemic diseases which killed the majority of all liveborn individuals before they reached maturity. On the highly speculative assumption that plague had returned to Europe in the eighteenth and early nineteenth centuries, one's guess – it can be no more – is that it might have had about the same significance as typhus and, like that disease, and all other infections, it would have responded to the major influences which transformed the health of the populations of the advanced countries in the past three centuries.

To summarize: micro-organisms and man have evolved in balance, and their relationship is constantly changing through the operation of natural selection in parasite and host. It is not to the advantage of

[8] J. F. D. Shrewsbury, *A History of Bubonic Plague in the British Isles.* Cambridge University Press (Cambridge, 1970), pp. 485–6.

[9] K. F. Helleiner, 'The vital revolution reconsidered.' *Canadian Journal of Economics and Political Science,* **23** (1957), pp. 1–9.

micro-organisms to kill their hosts, and after a period of adaptation the two may settle to a relation of mutual tolerance and, sometimes, advantage. However, disease or death may occur during the period of adaptation, or where the sickness of the hosts is necessary for the dissemination of the parasites. The stability of the relationship is different for different organisms; it is very variable in the case of the streptococcus, less so in that of the tubercle bacillus or measles virus. Changes in the character of infectious diseases of this type proceed continuously, and although related to the environment, are essentially independent of recognizable influences such as medical measures, hygiene and nutrition.

Although early man suffered from some infectious diseases, for example those contracted from animal vectors, living in small groups he is unlikely to have experienced many of the infections which were later prominent, particularly those which are airborne. The pattern of infectious diseases with which we are familiar probably dates from the domestication of plants and animals about 10,000 years ago, which led to the aggregation of populations of substantial size. The central problem of historical demography is to explain why the infections declined from the time of the modern agricultural and industrial revolutions, which led to still larger and more densely packed populations.

The decline of mortality from infectious diseases was not due substantially to a change in their character of the type defined above. Although there is no infection of which it can be said confidently that the relation between host and parasite has not varied over a specified period, this explanation is quite inadequate in the case of the airborne diseases. For to believe that the reduction of deaths was due essentially to a modification of their character, we should have to accept, either (a) that over a large range of airborne infections there was a favourable change of the kind which appears to have occurred in scarlet fever, independent of medical and other identifiable influences, or (b) that certain deleterious influences associated with industrialization led to high mortality in the eighteenth century which, through natural selection, resulted in the birth and survival of more resistant populations. The first explanation is frankly incredible, and the death rates of the eighteenth and early nineteenth centuries, particularly in Sweden, are inconsistent with the second. The same conclusion is suggested for water- and food-borne diseases, where the primary influence was clearly a reduction of exposure rather than an increase in the genetically determined resistance of those exposed. We cannot rule out the possibility of a change in the character of typhus, the only vector-borne disease which was significant in Britain after the beginning of the eighteenth century; but the contribution of the decline of this disease to the fall of mortality in the past three centuries was small.

Finally, I should emphasize that I have not concluded that there has been no change in the host/parasite relationship, except in the case of scarlet fever and a few other less clear-cut examples. On the contrary, it is possible that genetically determined resistance to diseases such as typhoid and tuberculosis is lower today than it was in the eighteenth and nineteenth centuries. But if so, this has come about as a secondary consequence of reduced exposure, rather than through a primary change in the relationship between organisms and man. Moreover, it is a change which, acting independently, would be expected to increase mortality rather than to reduce it.

5
The medical contribution

The conclusion that the decline of mortality from infectious diseases was not caused substantially by a change in their character leaves three other possibilities to be considered: a reduction of exposure to infection; increased general resistance due to improved nutrition; and prevention and treatment of the diseases by immunization and therapy. Although it might seem more logical to examine these influences in this order, because medical measures were long thought to be predominant they will be discussed first.

In addition to the natural immunity outlined in chapter 4, animals – in practice, usually man – can be protected by immunization and therapy. All that need be said about immunization by way of introduction is that while it protects against some infections, in general it is less effective than the protection afforded by experience of the disease itself. Not only is the immunity which results from immunization less effective; it is as a rule less durable. Medical treatment may also influence the course of infectious diseases by serum transfer, as in the treatment of diphtheria with antitoxin; or by therapy which acts directly on the micro-organism, as in the case of sulphonamides and antibiotics. There are other less specific clinical measures which are important in some cases, for example tracheotomy in laryngeal diphtheria, mechanical respiration in poliomyelitis and oxygen therapy in pneumonia.

Until recently it was accepted, almost without question, that the increase of population in the eighteenth century, and by inference later, was due to a decline of mortality brought about by medical advances. This conclusion was suggested by Talbot Griffith, who was impressed by developments in medicine in the eighteenth entury.[1] They included expansion of hospital, dispensary and midwifery services; notable

[1] G. T. Griffith, *Population Problems of the Age of Malthus.* Second edition, Frank Cass (London, 1967).

changes in medical education; advances in understanding of physiology and anatomy; and introduction of a specific protective measure, inoculation against smallpox. Taken together these developments seemed impressive, and it is scarcely surprising that Griffith, like most others who considered the matter, should have concluded that they contributed substantially to health. This conclusion, however, results from failure to distinguish clearly between the interests of the doctor and the interests of the patient, a common error in the interpretation of medical history. From the point of view of a student or practitioner of medicine, increased knowledge of anatomy, physiology and morbid anatomy are naturally regarded as important professional advances. But from the point of view of the patient, none of these changes has any practical significance until such time as it contributes to preservation of health or recovery from illness. It is because there is often a considerable interval between acquisition of new knowledge and any demonstrable benefit to the patient, that we cannot accept changes in medical education and institutions as evidence of the immediate effectiveness of medical measures. To arrive at a reliable opinion we must look critically at the work of doctors, and enquire whether in the light of present-day knowledge it is likely to have contributed significantly to the health of their patients.

The obvious way to do this is to assess the contribution which immunization and therapy have made to the control of the infectious diseases associated with the decline of mortality. Since this can be done reliably only from the time when cause of death was certified, I shall examine the influence of medical measures in the post-registration period before turning to the uncertainties of the eighteenth and early nineteenth centuries.

THE POST-REGISTRATION PERIOD

Airborne diseases (see table 3.2)

Tuberculosis   Figure 5.1 shows the trend of mortality from respiratory tuberculosis in England and Wales since 1838. This is the disease which, if any, was critical for the fall of the death rate. It was much the largest single cause of death in the mid-nineteenth century, and it was associated with nearly a fifth of the total reduction of mortality since then.

The time when effective medical measures became available is not in doubt. The tubercle bacillus was identified by Koch in 1882, but none of the treatments in use in the nineteenth or early twentieth century had a significant influence on the course of the disease. The many

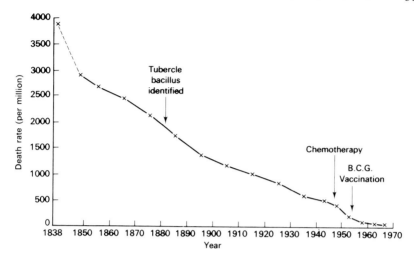

5.1 Respiratory tuberculosis: death rates, England and Wales.

chemotherapeutic agents that were tried are now known to have been ineffective, as was also the collapse therapy practised from about 1920. Effective treatment began with the introduction of streptomycin in 1947, and immunization (BCG vaccination) was used in England and Wales on a substantial scale from 1954. By these dates mortality from tuberculosis had fallen to a small fraction of its level in 1848–54; indeed most of the decline (57%) had taken place before the beginning of the present century. Nevertheless, there is no doubt about the contribution of chemotherapy, which was largely responsible for the rapid fall of mortality from the disease since 1950. Without this intervention the death rate would have continued to fall, but at a much slower rate.

Bronchitis, pneumonia and influenza   The trend of mortality from these diseases is shown in figure 5.2. The death rate increased in the second half of the nineteenth century but has fallen continuously, at least since the beginning of the twentieth. Although it is unfortunate that the limitations of national statistics make it necessary to consider the three diseases together, in relation to assessment of the effects of therapy this is not a serious disadvantage.

There is still no effective immunization against bronchitis and pneumonia. The influenza vaccines now available are not recommended for routine use or for the attempted control of outbreaks of the disease, so they have not influenced the trend of mortality. Therapy was useless before the introduction of the sulphonamides. The earliest (prontosil and sulphanilamide) were effective only against the strepto-

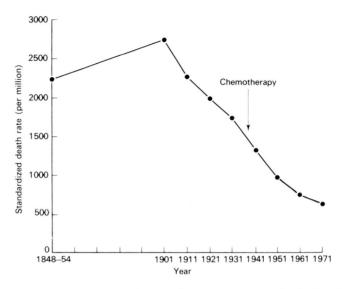

5.2 Bronchitis, pneumonia and influenza: death rates, England and Wales.

coccus, but trials of sulphapyridine in 1938 suggested that it reduced mortality from lobar pneumonia. Unfortunately it is difficult to assess the effect on mortality from national statistics, because of a change in the method of coding cause of death. (The method of selecting the primary cause of death when multiple causes were mentioned changed in 1940. Before then certain conditions were given an arbitrary order of preference according to the Registrar General's rules. From that time the primary cause was decided by the certifying practitioner. The effect of this change was small, except in the case of bronchitis which showed a large increase in the number of deaths, and diseases of the myocardium which showed a considerable decrease.) The picture is complicated further in the war period, when the data were based wholly on civilians, and when social conditions undoubtedly affected experience of respiratory diseases.

In view of these complications it is difficult, perhaps impossible, to assess precisely from when and to what extent therapeutic measures contributed to the reduction of mortality, particularly in the years following the introduction of sulphapyridine. What is clear is that this drug was not used until 1938 and was effective only in the treatment of lobar pneumonia. The scope of treatment was extended by the antibiotics which became available for civilian use in England and Wales from about the end of the Second World War.

Of the total decline of mortality between 1848–54 and 1971, bronchitis, pneumonia and influenza together contributed nearly a tenth (table 3.2); of the fall in the present century they contributed about a fifth.[2] Most of this decrease occurred before the introduction of sulphapyridine. There is no reason to doubt that the decline of mortality which started at the beginning of the century would have continued in the absence of effective therapeutic measures. Indeed in his address to the American Association of Immunologists in 1954, Magill noted that

> the rapid decline of pneumonia death rates began in New York State before the turn of the century and many years before the 'miracle drugs' were known. Certainly ... no-one ... has sufficient therapeutic faith to argue that the drugs available at the turn of the century were sufficiently potent to have initiated the precipitous drop in mortality. If we are disposed to be critical, we shall note that the steep downward trend in the pneumonia death rate began to taper off in the early 1940s, and that during the last few years the curve has followed a more or less horizontal course. It is of considerable interest that the initiation of that course of events coincided with the introduction of the antibiotics, and that the decline in the death rate essentially ceased as these agents became more and more universally employed.[3]

However, since there is both clinical and epidemiological evidence that sulphapyridine and the antibiotics are effective in treatment of the respiratory diseases, it would be accepted generally that they contributed to the subsequent reduction of mortality. Unfortunately, we cannot assess reliably the extent to which they did so; but it is clear that they were not responsible for all, or probably for most of the decrease which has occurred since 1938, and they can have had no influence on the substantial fall of deaths which occurred before that time.

Whooping cough   The trend of mortality from whooping cough is shown in figure 5.3, based on mean annual death rates of children under 15 in England and Wales. Mortality began to decline from the seventh decade of the nineteenth century, and the disease contributed 2·6 per cent to the reduction of the death rate from all causes.

Treatment by sulphonamides and, later, antibiotics was not available before 1938 and even now their effect on the course of the disease is questionable. Immunization was used widely after 1952; the protective effect is variable, and has been estimated to be between

[2] T. McKeown, R. G. Record and R. D. Turner, 'An interpretation of the decline of mortality in England and Wales during the twentieth century'. *Population Studies*, **29** (1975), p. 391.
[3] T. P. Magill, 'The immunologist and the evil spirits'. *Journal of Immunology*, **74** (1955), p. 1.

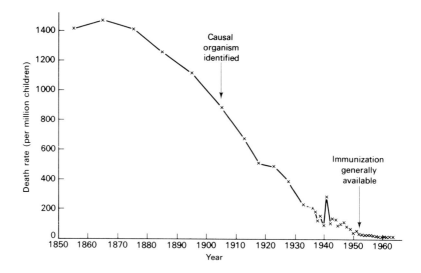

5.3 Whooping cough: death rates of children under 15, England and Wales.

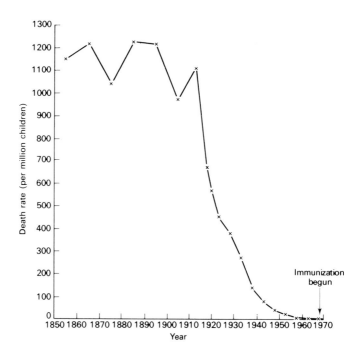

5.4 Measles: death rates of children under 15, England and Wales.

less than 20 and over 80 per cent. Clearly almost the whole of the decline of mortality from whooping cough occurred before the introduction of an effective medical measure.

Measles   Again the figure (5.4) is based on deaths of children under 15 in England and Wales. The picture is among the most remarkable for any infectious disease. Mortality fell rapidly and continuously from about 1915. Effective specific measures have only recently become available in the form of immunization, and they can have had no significant effect on the trend of the death rate. However, mortality from measles is due largely to invasion by secondary organisms, which have been treated by chemotherapy since 1935. Eighty-two per cent of the decrease of deaths from the disease occurred before this time.

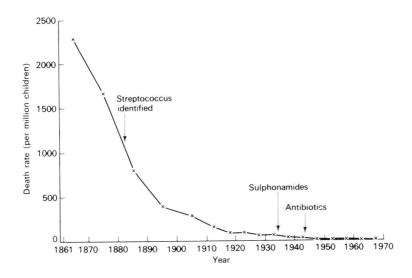

5.5 Scarlet fever: death rates of children under 15, England and Wales.

Scarlet fever   Because scarlet fever was grouped with diphtheria in the early years after registration of cause of death, the trend of mortality from the disease in children under 15 is shown from the seventh decade in figure 5.5. There was no effective treatment before the use of prontosil in 1935. But even by the beginning of the century mortality from scarlet fever had fallen to a relatively low level, and between 1901 and 1971 it was associated with only 1·2 per cent of the total reduction of the death rate from all causes. Approximately 90 per cent of this improvement occurred before the use of the sulphonamides.

Diphtheria Figure 5.6 is based on the mean annual death rate of children under 15, from the eighth decade of the nineteenth century. It is perhaps the infectious disease in which it is most difficult to assess precisely the time and influence of therapeutic measures. Antitoxin was used first in the late nineteenth century and has been the accepted form of treatment since then. It is believed to have reduced the case fatality rate, which fell from 8·2 per 100 notifications in 1916–25 to 5·4 in 1933–42, while notifications remained at an average level of about 50,000 per year. The mortality rate increased at the beginning of the last war but fell rapidly at about the time when national immunization began.

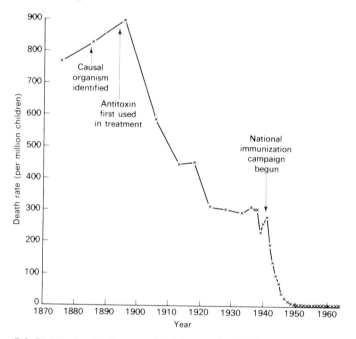

5.6 Diphtheria: death rates of children under 15, England and Wales.

It is tempting to attribute much of the decline of diphtheria mortality between 1900 and 1931 to treatment by antitoxin and the rapid fall since 1941 to immunization. Nothing in British experience is seriously inconsistent with this interpretation. However, experience in some other countries is not so impressive; for example there are American States where the reduction of mortality in the 1940s did not coincide with the immunization programme. Moreover, several other infections, particularly those that are airborne, declined in the same period in the absence of effective prophylaxis or treatment. While therefore it is usual, and probably reasonable, to attribute the fall of mortality from diphtheria in this century largely to medical measures, we cannot exclude the possibility that other influences also contributed, perhaps substantially.

Smallpox The death rate from smallpox in the mid-nineteenth century was a good deal smaller than that of the infections already discussed, and the somewhat erratic trend of mortality since then is shown in figure 5.7. Vaccination of infants was made compulsory in 1854 but the law was not enforced until 1871. From that time until 1898, when

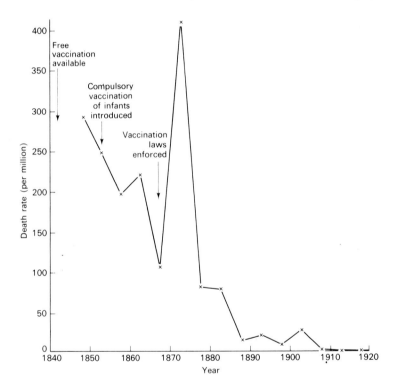

5.7 Smallpox: death rates, England and Wales.

the conscientious objector's clause was introduced, almost all children were vaccinated. The relative importance of mass vaccination and of surveillance followed by vaccination of contacts was referred to in the opening chapter. However, most epidemiologists are agreed that we owe the decline of mortality from smallpox mainly to vaccination. Since the mid-nineteenth century the decrease has been associated with only 1·6 per cent of the reduction of the death rate from all causes.

Infections of ear, pharynx and larynx   Together these diseases also were associated with only a small part (0·8 per cent) of the decrease of deaths. The main therapeutic influences have been chemotherapy and, in some ear infections, surgery. It is difficult to give a time from which surgical intervention can be said to have been beneficial, but in view of the small contribution made by these diseases it is perhaps not very important to assess it more precisely than by saying that one third of the decline (0·3 per cent of mortality from all causes in this century) occurred before the use of sulphonamides in 1935.

Poliomyelitis   Before completing this assessment of the contribution of immunization and therapy to the control of airborne infections, I should refer to poliomyelitis, whose prevention by vaccination is widely regarded as one of the triumphs of modern medicine. It appears to have been a rare disease before the late nineteenth century, but since that time it has occurred in epidemics in many countries. It is due to a virus which infects the alimentary tract but only occasionally causes the paralysis which is a striking feature of the disease; the number of persons infected but with few or no clinical manifestations exceeds greatly the number affected by paralysis. In its paralytic form poliomyelitis presents the anomaly of an intestinal infection whose incidence increases as social conditions improve, for it is most common in countries with a high standard of living. An explanation usually offered is that in primitive conditions children acquire immunity by early exposure to the infection (the polio virus is endemic in communities with poor hygiene), whereas if hygiene is good they are protected from exposure and hence less resistant when they meet the disease in adult life. It is consistent with this interpretation that although the disease is most common in young children, its clinical manifestations are more severe in adults.

Because of the conspicuous disabilities which occur in patients who survive, there is, understandably, some tendency to overestimate the significance of poliomyelitis in relation to other infections. In 1947 there were 33 deaths from the disease per million children under 15, compared with 99 from whooping cough and 69 from measles. In 1871–80, before the decline of mortality began, the last two diseases were responsible for 1415 and 1038 deaths (per million under 15) respectively.

Poliomyelitis was recognized as an infection in 1909 and shown to be due to a filterable virus. Two methods of immunization have been used widely: inactivated vaccine containing killed virus (Salk); and live attenuated virus vaccine (Sabin). The former was in use in Britain from 1956, but the latter is generally preferred, since it can be given orally and the immunity conferred is greater and lasts longer.

Immunization became common in England and Wales in 1956.

Before this time mortality from poliomyelitis varied considerably from year to year and it is impossible to assess accurately the contribution of vaccination. Nevertheless there are grounds for believing that it was very effective, both from the laboratory and from controlled clinical trials. The disease has been almost eliminated from countries which have had effective immunization programmes, whereas it is still common in countries which have not. But of course in relation to the total decline of mortality from all causes, the reduction associated with poliomyelitis was very small.

In summary, the airborne diseases accounted for two fifths of the reduction of mortality from all causes from the mid nineteenth century to 1971. Vaccination against smallpox was the only medical measure which contributed to the fall of deaths before 1900, and this disease was associated with only a small part (1·6 per cent) of the decrease of the death rate from all causes. In this century antitoxin probably lowered mortality from diphtheria, and surgery may have reduced deaths from ear infections, but together these influences had little effect on total deaths. With these exceptions, effective medical intervention began with the chemotherapeutic agents which became available after 1935, particularly the sulphonamides and antibiotics. By this time mortality from airborne infections had fallen to a small fraction of its level in the mid-nineteenth century; and even after the introduction of chemotherapy, with the important exception of tuberculosis, it is probably safe to conclude that immunization and therapy were not the main influences on the further decline of the death rate.

Water- and food-borne diseases (see table 3.3)

Cholera, diarrhoea and dysentery   In the mid-nineteenth century cholera was grouped with other diarrhoeal diseases in the Registrar General's classification; however, the last epidemic in Britain was in 1865, so from that time the contribution of cholera was negligible. Mortality from the diarrhoeal diseases fell in the late nineteenth century; it increased between 1901 and 1911 but then decreased rapidly.

It is unlikely that treatment had any appreciable effect on the outcome of the diseases before the use of intravenous therapy in the nineteen thirties, by which time 95 per cent of the improvement had occurred. For the main explanation of the decline of mortality we must turn to the hygienic measures which reduced exposure. They will be discussed in the next chapter.

Non-respiratory tuberculosis   Non-respiratory tuberculosis was an important cause of death in the nineteenth century. Although mortality fell quite rapidly after 1901, there was still a considerable number of deaths in England and Wales (197) in 1971.

Interpretation of this trend is complicated by the fact that non-respiratory tuberculosis is due to both human and bovine infections; the abdominal cases are predominantly of bovine origin, whereas those involving other organs such as bones are often caused by the human organism. The human types can be interpreted in the same terms as the pulmonary disease, but a different explanation must be sought for the bovine infection. It is unlikely that treatment contributed significantly to the fall of mortality, since the level was already low when streptomycin – the first effective measure – was introduced in 1947.

Typhoid and typhus As noted in chapter 3, mortality from typhus fell rapidly in the late nineteenth century and there have been few deaths in the twentieth. It can be said without hesitation that specific medical measures had no influence on this decline.

The decline of the enteric fevers was also rapid, and began before the turn of the century, somewhat earlier than the fall of deaths from diarrhoea and dysentery. Effective treatment by chloramphenicol was not available until 1950, but by that time mortality from enteric fever was almost eliminated from England and Wales. Although immunization was used widely in the armed services during the war, its effectiveness is doubtful and it can have had little influence on the number of deaths.

In summary, the rapid decline of mortality from the diseases spread by water and food since the late nineteenth century owed little to medical measures. Immunization is relatively ineffective even today, and therapy of some value was not employed until about 1950, by which time the number of deaths had fallen to a very low level.

Other diseases due to micro-organisms (see table 3.4)

Convulsions and teething As mentioned in chapter 3, most of the deaths included under these unsatisfactory terms were due to infectious diseases of childhood, for example to whooping cough, measles, otitis media, meningitis and gastro-enteritis. These infections are mainly airborne, and the general conclusions concerning the time and influence of immunization and therapy on airborne diseases may be accepted for them. That is to say, it is unlikely that medical measures had any significant effect on the frequency of death before the introduction of sulphonamides and antibiotics, and even after that time they were probably less important than other influences.

Syphilis   Although syphilis was associated with only 0·3 per cent of the reduction of mortality from the mid-nineteenth century to 1971, it remained an important cause of sickness and death until about 1916, when salvarson was made available free of charge to medical practitioners. From this time the number of deaths fell, and it was quite low in 1945 when penicillin largely replaced the arsenical preparations.

The decline of syphilis since its introduction to Europe in the fifteenth century was not due mainly to therapy, for after several centuries of exposure of the population the disease had changed to a milder form. Nevertheless it seems reasonable to attribute the reduction of mortality since 1901 essentially to treatment. It should of course be recognized that effective treatment, as in the case of tuberculosis, not only benefits those affected by the disease, but also reduces the number of persons who spread the infection. It seems right to regard this secondary effect as a further contribution of medical measures.

Appendicitis, peritonitis   Mortality from these causes increased slightly during the nineteenth and early twentieth centuries – probably because of more accurate certification of cause of death – but declined after 1921. This improvement, which accounted for 0·4 per cent of the fall of death rate from all causes, can be attributed to treatment.

Puerperal fever   The death rate from puerperal fever declined from the beginning of this century, but more rapidly after the introduction of the sulphonamides (1935) and, later, penicillin. It seems probable that the initial fall was due mainly to reduced exposure to infection, as the teaching of Semmelweis in the previous century began to improve the practice of the developing midwifery services; but from 1935 these services were greatly reinforced by chemotherapy. Both influences can be credited to medical interventions.

Other infections   The 'other conditions' shown in table 3.4 are a miscellaneous group, including some well recognized infectious diseases which caused few deaths, either because they were uncommon in this period (as in the case of malaria, tetanus, poliomyelitis and encephalitis) or because although common they were not often lethal (as in the case of mumps, chicken pox and rubella). They also include some relatively uncommon certified causes of death which are ill defined, such as abscess, phlegmon and pyaemia. In addition there is a very small number of deaths due to worm parasites which, strictly, do not belong among conditions due to micro-organisms.

These infections were associated with 3·5 per cent of the fall of mortality between the mid-nineteenth century and 1971. In view of their varied aetiology it is not possible to assess accurately the major influences, but it is unlikely that therapy made much contribution before 1935. More than half of the reduction of deaths occurred before this time.

THE EIGHTEENTH AND EARLY NINETEENTH CENTURIES

From the conclusion that immunization and therapy had little influence on the trend of mortality from infectious diseases in the hundred years after registration of cause of death, it would seem to follow that they are very unlikely to have contributed significantly in the century that preceded it. Some historians who, like Griffith, concluded that medical measures were important in the eighteenth century, were clearly unaware that they have had a relatively small effect on the death rate even to the present day; but there are others who have taken the same position in the face of evidence that it is inconsistent with recent experience.

The most satisfactory way to assess the contribution of immunization and therapy would be the one adopted for the post-registration period, namely to examine their effects on the diseases associated with the decline of mortality. However this approach requires knowledge of cause of death which is not available for the eighteenth century, so one must rely on a general appraisal of the medical advances of that time.

The discussion which follows is based on the conclusions reached by McKeown and Brown, extended, in the case of inoculation, in the light of more recent experience.[4] Midwifery services are considered as a whole in this context, because although they may also influence non-infective conditions, their impact in the eighteenth and early nineteenth centuries would have been chiefly on infectious causes of maternal and infant deaths.

Midwifery

To assess the effect of midwifery on mortality we must consider two important changes in obstetric practice during the eighteenth century: the introduction on a substantial scale of institutional delivery; and a change in obstetric technique and management which possibly had its main impact on domiciliary practice.

Before 1749, when the first lying-in hospital was founded in London, institutional delivery was very uncommon. A considerable number of lying-in hospitals were established during the second half of the eighteenth century, and Griffith included them among 'notable improvements during the period'.[5] But when first introduced, and for

[4] T. McKeown and R. G. Brown, 'Medical evidence related to English population changes in the eighteenth century'. *Population Studies*, **9** (1955), p. 119.

[5] *Population Problems of the Age of Malthus, op. cit.*

many years after, the practice of institutional confinement had an adverse effect on mortality.

During the 13 years from 1855 to 1867, there were 4·83 maternal deaths per thousand deliveries in England. Results of institutional and domiciliary delivery were quite different. Lefort estimated mortality in a large number of confinements in all parts of Europe as 34 and 4·7 per thousand deliveries for institutional and domiciliary deliveries respectively; contemporary English estimates were consistent with these figures.[6] There was substantial variation in the rates from one hospital to another, and in the same hospital from year to year, but with few exceptions hospital death rates were many times greater than those for related home deliveries. Indeed the difference was so conspicuous that it was obvious to contemporary observers, and Ericksen noted that 'a woman has a better chance of recovery after delivery in the meanest, poorest hovel, than in the best conducted general hospital, furnished with every appliance that can add to her comfort, and with the best skill that a metropolis can afford.'[7] There is of course no mystery about the reason for the high death rates; most deaths were due to puerperal infection.

The figures quoted are from the mid-nineteenth century, and it may be asked whether results of institutional delivery at the earlier period were equally bad. There is reason to believe that they were worse. National statistics are not, of course, available, but from records of individual hospitals it seems probable that results were slightly better in the nineteenth century than in the last quarter of the eighteenth. There can be little doubt that the effect of institutional confinement on maternal mortality was wholly bad, and indeed had the proportion of deliveries conducted in hospitals approached that in some modern communities, the results would have been reflected in national statistics.

I must now enquire whether changes in obstetric technique and management contributed to a reduction of mortality. During the second half of the century delivery by forceps and other artificial means became more common, and the formidable instruments in earlier use had been modified to some extent. Data quoted by Simpson and others show that even in hospital practice, delivery by forceps was unusual (a few cases in every thousand deliveries) and results on the mortality of mother and child were extremely bad.[8] For example, in a Dublin series the proportion of deaths after operative or artificial delivery was approximately 3 in 4 for children and 1 in 4 for mothers. Even if artificial delivery was relatively more common in home confinements, which is unlikely, and if results were much better than in hospital,

[6] L. Lefort, *Des Maternités.* (Paris, 1866.)

[7] J. E. Ericksen, *On Hospitalism and the Causes of Death after Operations.* (London, 1874.)

[8] J. Y. Simpson, *Obstetric Memoirs and Contributions,* vol. 1. (Edinburgh, 1855), pp. 626, 855.

which is quite possible, it seems inconceivable that the use of instruments had a favourable effect on obstetric practice.

Much more significant was a change in the conditions under which deliveries were conducted. This was not so much a variation in obstetric technique as an improvement of hygiene in the labour room. White, for example, recommended cleanliness and adequate ventilation, and claimed that by having regard to these essentials he had lost no patients because of puerperal infection.[9] It is not known how widely such practices were followed in domiciliary obstetrics in the late eighteenth century, and it must be remembered that many years later it was by no means generally accepted, even by medical practitioners, that the environment contributed to ill health. Nevertheless it is possible that maternal mortality fell during the eighteenth century, and the simple hygienic measures practised by White and others may be the most important contribution which doctors made to this improvement.

I have so far examined the influence of midwifery on maternal mortality. Today in most western countries maternal mortality is so low that the mortality of the foetus or newborn infant provides a more sensitive index of the effectiveness of an obstetric service. But in the eighteenth and nineteenth centuries high infant death rates were generally regarded as inevitable, and infant mortality rates were not given in national statistics until 1841, nor stillbirth rates until 1927. Nevertheless, there seems no reason to doubt that the conclusions which emerge from consideration of maternal mortality would be confirmed if statistics on foetal and infant deaths were available. These conclusions are: that the introduction of institutional confinement had an adverse effect on mortality – newborn infants are even more vulnerable than their mothers to infectious disease and mortality rates in hospital were consistently higher than in domiciliary practice; and that the only change in obstetric practice likely to have contributed to a reduction of maternal or infant mortality was an improvement in the hygiene of delivery.

Medicines
The only drugs available in the eighteenth century which might conceivably have had a significant influence on deaths from infectious diseases are mercury and cinchona in the treatment of syphilis and malaria. Mercury was introduced during the late fifteenth century, largely abandoned during the sixteenth and seventeenth centuries, and reintroduced during the eighteenth. This drug is no longer used by itself, although until recently it was valued as a therapeutic agent in treatment of syphilis. But while mercury may have had some effect

[9] C. White, *A Treatise on the Management of Pregnant and Lying-in Women.* (1773.)

upon the course of the disease in individual cases, it is hard to believe that its influence can have been reflected in national mortality rates.

Cinchona was known in England from about 1655 and was listed in the London Pharmacopeia in 1677. It is undoubtedly effective in the treatment of malaria; but during most of the eighteenth century cinchona was given in doses which were too small to be really effective, until Lind demonstrated in 1786 that large doses were essential. It was also used indiscriminately, since malaria was not identified clearly from other fevers. Moreover, the number of deaths attributed to ague was insignificant in relation to the total death rate; according to Blane there were 44 deaths in the bills of mortality in 1728, and only 16 in 1730.[10]

Inoculation

In the opening chapter I referred to the suggestion that inoculation was effective in preventing smallpox in the eighteenth century, and that it made a substantial contribution to the reduction of deaths and growth of population.[11] This conclusion was rejected in a recent review of the history of smallpox:

> Here was the fundamental weakness of the procedure of variolation. Its objective was not to prevent smallpox, but to induce artificially – at a chosen time when the subject was in good health, and by using matter from a mild case – a mild attack of the disease that would confer protection against a more serious naturally acquired attack. Although there were many successes there were also many failures in the form of fatal infections. Moreover, variolation was sometimes responsible for local epidemics of smallpox. A Dr R. Willan reported that in 1796 one variolated child had infected 17 persons with smallpox, of whom 8 died. From such evidence as is available it seems clear that variolation tended rather to increase than to decrease the incidence of smallpox.[12]

Among reasons given in the opening chapter for rejecting the conclusion that variolation reduced mortality from smallpox, was the observation that control of the disease has been achieved by surveillance and vaccination of contacts rather than by mass immunization. The summary which follows is based on the extensive and worldwide experience of the World Health Organization:

> Early in the smallpox eradication campaign, it was realized that

[10] G. Blane, 'Observations on the comparative prevalence, mortality and treatment of different diseases'. *Medico-Chirurgical Transactions*, **4** (1813), p. 94.

[11] P. E.Razzell, 'Population change in eighteenth century England; a reinterpretation'. *Economic History Review* (2nd series), **18** (1965), p. 312.

[12] N. Howard-Jones, 'Thousand-year scourge'. *World Health* (February–March, 1975), pp. 7–8.

vaccination of everyone in a population was impossible. Migrants, field workers and those living in congested slums frequently were missed or evaded vaccination – and every day children were born. Even when the vast majority had been immunized, the virus continued to smoulder among those still susceptible. Fundamental to the complete conquest of the disease is the understanding that only a small pocket of poorly protected persons can set smallpox raging again. But even where only a minority have been vaccinated, a good surveillance system to detect cases – coupled with vigorous containment measures – can cut the deadly chain of transmission and thereby vanquish the disease.

As they gained experience in the war against variola, national health armies changed battle plans, shifting their heaviest guns from trying to vaccinate 'everyone' to the strategy of surveillance – followed by quick containment and elimination of the outbreak. At first, while smallpox was common, this strategy enabled broader inroads to be made against contagion; later, it permitted efficient countermeasures against reintroduction of smallpox and, finally, it was effective in verifying that the disease had indeed been banished.

In several countries, transmission of smallpox was halted less than one year after surveillance programmes had become established, despite the fact that by no means all their citizens had been vaccinated. In other countries, where mass vaccination alone was attempted, but was unaccompanied by adequate surveillance and containment, smallpox persisted.[13]

In the light of this experience it is most unlikely that inoculation had a significant influence on the national death rate in the eighteenth century, nearly a hundred years before the discovery of micro-organisms, and a century and a half earlier than the first specific measure which, had it been available, might possibly have had such an effect. I refer to streptomycin in treatment of tuberculosis.

To summarize: except in the case of vaccination against smallpox (which was associated with 1·6 per cent of the decline of the death rate from 1848–54 to 1971), it is unlikely that immunization or therapy had a significant effect on mortality from infectious diseases before the twentieth century. Between 1900 and 1935 these measures contributed in some diseases: antitoxin in treatment of diphtheria; surgery in treatment of appendicitis, peritonitis and ear infections; salvarsan in treatment of syphilis; intravenous therapy in treatment of diarrhoeal diseases; passive immunization against tetanus; and improved obstetric care resulting in prevention of puerperal fever. But even if these

[13] J. Klein, 'A strategy of surveillance'. *Smallpox: Point of No Return* (1975), World Health Day, 75/5.

measures were responsible for the whole decline of mortality from these conditions after 1900 – which clearly they were not – they would account for only a very small part of the decrease of deaths which occurred before 1935. From that time the first powerful chemotherapeutic agents – sulphonamides and, later, antibiotics – came into use, and they were supplemented by improved vaccines. However, they were certainly not the only influences which led to the continued fall of mortality. I conclude that immunization and treatment contributed little to the reduction of deaths from infectious diseases before 1935, and over the whole period since cause of death was first registered (in 1838) they were much less important than other influences.

It would be surprising if medical measures were more effective in the period which preceded registration of cause of death than in the century which followed. Although the diseases which declined in the eighteenth and early nineteenth century cannot be examined individually, appraisal of medical developments – in midwifery, medicines and inoculation – suggests that they had no significant effect on the trend of mortality and growth of population.

6
Exposure to infection

MODES OF SPREAD OF MICRO-ORGANISMS

From the outset it is clear that at least part of the decline of mortality from infectious diseases was due to reduced contact with micro-organisms. In the so-called developed countries an individual no longer meets the cholera vibrio, he is rarely exposed to the typhoid organism and he is infected by the tubercle bacillus much less often than in the past. But, so far as can be judged, there has been no large change in frequency of exposure to the streptococcus or the measles virus, so we must look elsewhere for an explanation of the decline of deaths from scarlet fever and measles.

The feasibility of preventing contact with micro-organisms is determined largely by the ways they are spread. There are five main routes: by water, food, animal vectors, air and personal contact.

Water-borne diseases
With some exceptions the major water-borne diseases are spread by contamination of water with infected human faeces or urine. The organisms may reach the host in drinking water or from water in contact with the skin.

Cholera is an example of an infectious disease spread through faecal contamination of drinking water, although it can also be acquired from infected food and by direct contact. Typhoid fever, the other major water-borne infectious disease of which the developed countries have had considerable experience, is transmitted in the same way. So, too, is amoebic dysentery.

The most important disease which reaches the host from water through the skin is schistosomiasis. It is widespread in Africa, Latin America and the Far East, and threatens to displace malaria in international importance. It is found wherever man comes into barefooted contact with water suitable for the appropriate species of snails. The adult worms live in the human portal system and pelvic veins and the eggs are excreted in the urine and faeces. In water the eggs hatch and the trematode continues its developmental cycle in the tissues of the snail vector, from which it again enters the water to gain access to a human host through the unbroken skin. The disease is formidably difficult to control and irrigation schemes are introducing it into new areas.

Weil's disease is an example of the less common transmission by water of micro-organisms excreted by other animals. The causal organism (Leptospira icterohaemorrhagica) is excreted in the urine of infected rats and can survive for several weeks in water, from which it enters the human host through the skin. As a result of its mode of spread, Weil's disease is associated with occupations such as farming, coal mining, work in sewers and fish handling, which bring workers into contact with rat-infested waters.

Food-borne diseases
Many bacterial and some viral and parasitic diseases are transmitted by contaminated food. Sometimes the food comes from infected animals (poultry, swine and cattle with salmonella and cattle with tuberculosis and brucellosis), or from animals living in infected water (oysters and mussels which transmit typhoid); but the pathogen may be introduced into food by someone carrying infection (dysentery, typhoid and paratyphoid) or by contaminated water.

In the past milk was probably the most important vehicle for food-borne disease. It forms an excellent culture medium for many pathogens and was responsible for outbreaks of dysentery, typhoid and paratyphoid fever, streptococcal sore throat and infantile gastro-enteritis. Milk from infected animals was the source of bone, joint and glandular tuberculosis and brucellosis. Abdominal tuberculosis in children under 15 was usually due to infected milk, and mortality from this condition provided a good index of the amount of bovine tuberculosis. Young children are particularly susceptible to bowel infection from contaminated milk, and infant mortality from diarrhoea was much less common among breast fed children than in those fed in other ways.

Many of the worms which parasitize man are transmitted by food. The tapeworms Taenia saginata and Taenia solium have cattle and pigs as intermediate hosts. Gravid segments of the worm are passed in the stools of infected persons, and the eggs, if swallowed by the appropriate animal vector, liberate embryos which find their way into the skeletal muscles where they encyst. The worm is acquired by eating the muscles raw or incompletely cooked. Man sometimes becomes involved in the life cycle of the small tapeworm Echinococcus granulosus, of which the common definitive host is the dog and the usual intermediate host is the sheep. Hydatid disease results from ingesting the eggs excreted by infected dogs; it is common in some parts of the world and still occurs from time to time in Britain.

Animal-borne diseases

It is difficult to exaggerate the importance of other animals, arthropods as well as vertebrates, as reservoirs and transmitters of human disease. The rat with its fleas has carried bubonic plague in epidemics since the beginning of history. The body louse has been responsible for more deaths of soldiers from typhus than all the weapons of mankind. Mosquitoes, by transmitting malaria and yellow fever and tsetse flies by transmitting trypanosomiasis have depopulated millions of square miles of fertile land. Even today animal-borne diseases are so widespread and so debilitating that they profoundly depress productivity in a world chronically short of food. More than a hundred of the communicable diseases affecting man have animal links in their chains of transmission. All the known infective agents are implicated (viruses, rickettsiae, bacteria, fungi, protozoa and helminths); the animal vectors include all the common domestic animals and many wild vertebrates, as well as insects and molluscs. The way in which the diseases are transmitted is of great importance in relation to control.

A number of diseases are acquired by direct physical contact with infected animals or their carcasses. Rabies is transmitted to man by infected dogs, cats or, in parts of America, vampire bats; the main source of human anthrax is contact with the carcasses, wool, hair or hides of animals or with feeding stuffs and fertilizers made from their bodies, Orf, cowpox, rat-bite fever and certain of the dermatomycoses (cat, dog, cattle and horse ringworm) are other examples of diseases transmitted directly by infected animals.

Much more important are the infections transmitted indirectly through animal intermediaries or vectors (vertebrate and invertebrate). The modes of transmission are varied and often complex. The vector may act only as a mechanical vehicle which carries the parasite from one host to another. In this way flies transfer the organisms of bacillary dysentery from infected faeces to food and cooking utensils, although transmission usually results from close person-to-person association. More often the vector is involved biologically. For example, the rickettsiae of typhus multiply in the cells of the louse midgut; the louse defaecates as it bites and the human host is inoculated with the infected faeces when he scratches. Sometimes the animal vector plays an essential part in the life cycle of the parasite; the sexual cycle of the malaria protozoon takes place only in anopheline mosquitoes. Or several animal intermediaries may be involved before a new human host becomes infected: for example, the adult fish tapeworm Diphyllobothrium latum inhabits the human intestine; the eggs are excreted with the faeces, and in fresh water produce free-swimming larvae; the larvae enter the next phase of their development when ingested by crustaceans; they undergo further development when the crustaceans are swallowed by small fish; when the fish are swallowed by larger fish, the larvae invade and become encysted in the muscles of the new hosts; the cycle is completed when man eats the raw, smoked or pickled flesh of the infected fish.

The nature of the animal vector (arthropod, mollusc or vertebrate) has an important bearing on control of the indirectly transmitted infections. Malaria, yellow fever, typhus and trypanosomiasis are all transmitted by arthropod vectors.

Malaria is conveyed only by anopheline mosquitoes. The sporozoites find their way into the insect's salivary glands, from which they are injected into the human blood stream when the female mosquito is feeding. The clinical features of the disease are determined by the species of plasmodium involved, and its epidemiological pattern by the habits of fifty or more species of anopheline vectors. All depend upon water for their larval stage, but the choice of water (clean, brackish, tidal, sunlit, shady), flight range, feeding habits and resting place vary from species to species. Climatic conditions are also important; a temperature of at least 20° is required before the sexual cycle of Plasmodium falciparum (the cause of malignant subtertian malaria) can be completed in the mosquito and a temperature of 15°C is needed for other species. For this reason it is unlikely that malaria was ever common in Britain, since the required temperature is not maintained for long enough to support the life cycle of the parasite. Nevertheless the disease can be transmitted; for example in the years which followed the First World War, 359 cases were notified in Kent, the infection having been carried by anophelines in the Thames marshes.

Yellow fever, a virus disease, is also conveyed by mosquitoes. In its epidemic form it is confined to man and transmitted only by Aëdes aegypti, a domestic moquito which breeds in small collections of rain water, such as may be found in a discarded tin or the bottom of a boat. Since this mosquito requires for its life cycle a mean temperature of at least 24°C, it is confined to the tropics. Although the vector is common in Asia and the Pacific, yellow fever is seen only in Africa and South America. In endemic form (jungle yellow fever) the disease occurs sporadically in scattered rural communities of tropical rain forests. This form of the disease has its reservoir in certain species of monkeys and is transmitted from them to man by mosquitoes.

Typhus fevers, due to infection with rickettsiae, are transmitted by many different arthropods – lice, fleas, ticks and mites. There appears to be no animal reservoir of epidemic typhus, which in previous centuries was the destroyer of armies and the scrouge of hospitals and prisons. The disease is transmitted from man to man by the body louse, which usually dies from the infection. The many other typhus fevers are primarily animal infections, transferred from animal to animal by arthropods and occasionally conveyed to man by the bites of the vectors. Murine typhus is a world wide infection of rats, sporadically transmitted by infected rat fleas. Dogs and rodents are also subject to tick-borne typhus infections, occasionally conveyed to man, as in the cases of Rocky Mountain spotted fever and north Queensland and Kenya typhus.

African trypanosomiasis is transmitted by the bite of the tsetse fly, which is biologically involved in the developmental cycle of the protozoon. The different species of the vector are often very specific in their environmental needs, some surviving only near rivers and streams, others requiring shrubs and trees in scrub and bush country. In consequence the human form of the disease, sleeping sickness, is essentially a rural disease, for the vectors cannot survive in an urban environment. Trypanosomiasis of cattle (ngana) has delayed the development of vast tracts of good grazing land in central Africa and is indirectly of considerable medical importance because of its effect upon human nutrition.

Airborne diseases

Airborne infections are spread in two main ways: directly from one individual to another by droplets or droplet nuclei; and indirectly by dust from bedding, clothes, carpets and floors. The methods are not necessarily disease specific; for example smallpox, pulmonary tuberculosis and streptococcal infections are transmitted by droplet nuclei, but also, less frequently, by dust. Some infections that are normally airborne (streptococcal sore throat and diphtheria) may be spread by contamination of food, usually milk.

During quiet breathing few droplets are expelled; they are produced by talking, and in much greater numbers by coughing and sneezing. The largest droplets fall rapidly to the ground or on to the clothes or bedding of the person producing them. Droplets of less than 100 μm in diameter descend more slowly, evaporating as they fall. Depending upon their size, atmospheric humidity, air movement and other influences, a proportion of these smaller droplets lose all their moisture before they reach the ground and remain suspended as droplet nuclei until removed by ventilation. It follows that for infection to be transmitted by droplet spray the susceptible host needs to be very near the source of infection; a child standing close to an infected person is particularly vulnerable. Diseases disseminated mainly by this method are often associated with overcrowded sleeping conditions, as in the case of cerebrospinal meningitis among service personnel, or with close family contact, as in the case of whooping cough. Droplet nuclei, on the other hand, because they remain airborne, transmit infection over much greater distances. The viruses of measles and chicken pox are readily disseminated in this way. Because of their small size and low settling velocity the nuclei are carried into the alveoli of the lungs, and it is therefore possible for a susceptible person to become infected from the inhalation of a very small number.

When large droplets fall to the ground they dry out and become part of the dust of the room. If they contain pathogens resistant to drying, the dust may act as a reservoir of infection for a long time (tubercle bacilli have been known to survive in dust for three months and haemolytic streptococci for six months). Organisms from soiled surgical dressings, skin scales, dried sputum and other secretions may also become part of the dust of a room, and cross-infection in surgical wards is often traced to these sources. However, except in places such as hospitals, dust is not a common vehicle for transmission of airborne infections; for although huge numbers of particles containing living organisms become airborne when the dust in a room is disturbed by domestic activities, most of the organisms are not pathogenic.

Diseases spread by personal contact
Most micro-organisms which are spread from man to man are transmitted by one or more of the routes described above and this section is concerned only with diseases which are caused by human physical contact, direct or indirect. Within this class it will be unnecessary to consider diseases whose transmission is autogenous, that is to say which are spread from one part of the body (naso-pharynx, intestinal tract, ano-genital region, skin and anterior nares) to another part of the same individual. Diseases which remain after these exclusions include venereal infections, scabies, ringworm, impetigo, leprosy, yaws and trachoma, of which the last three are confined to tropical countries. Although these diseases cause a good deal of morbidity they are not now, and with the exception of syphilis were not in the past, responsible for much mortality.

FEASIBILITY OF CONTROL OF TRANSMISSION

Against the background of the preceding discussion it is possible to assess the feasibility of control of spread of micro-organisms according to their modes of transmission. It is important to consider separately technologically advanced countries, located usually in temperate zones, and developing countries, mainly in tropical or sub-tropical areas.

In advanced countries there is little doubt that the infectious diseases most readily controlled by hygienic measures are those spread by water. Their prevention requires mainly purification of water supplies and efficient sewage disposal, and it is significant that throughout the western world these were the first important advances in the control of the physical environment. Given the necessary resources, these measures can be introduced quickly, and do not require for their effectiveness the cooperation of the individual from day to day. Nevertheless the problems have not all been solved, for there is still serious pollution of rivers and seas from sewage effluents.

It is more difficult to control the cleanliness of food, for the conditions under which food is prepared, stored, distributed and eaten depend largely on individual actions. Hence, while infection from water is very unusual in developed countries, single cases of food poisoning are relatively common and there are occasional outbreaks affecting considerable numbers of people.

It is still more difficult to prevent diseases spread by direct personal contact. Since their transmission is determined by personal behaviour and hygiene, it might be thought that they would be controlled readily in literate populations with a reasonable standard of living. This is true of scabies, ringworm and impetigo; it is not true of venereal infections, in which appeals for continence or for contraceptive measures which prevent disease as well as conception have not had much effect. Indeed the use of the pill has probably increased the frequency of exposure to venereally transmitted disease, because it has encouraged promiscuity without reducing the likelihood of infection.

Among diseases spread by animal vectors we are concerned with those transmitted directly by animals (usually by a bite), and not with others conveyed indirectly from animals through media such as water and food. Some of the diseases in the former class (for example anthrax and rabies) are relatively uncommon; the important ones are transmitted by arthropods – fleas, lice, flies and mosquitoes. These vectors vary widely in the feasibility of their control. Some (the fleas and lice responsible for the transmission of typhus fever) seem to disappear with a rising standard of living. Others (anopheline mosquitoes) are susceptible to modern insecticides. Still others, such as the common house fly, can be contained but not eliminated, by stringent hygiene, both public and private.

However, it is the airborne infections which present the most formidable problems. There are broadly two ways in which control of their spread may be attempted: by removing the source of the infection, usually by isolating from the community those suffering from or possibly incubating an infection; and by interrupting lines of communication, by ventilation and prevention of overcrowding. But these measures have relatively little effect on exposure of a population to most airborne infections. They have had no substantial influence on the spread of diseases such as measles, whooping cough and scarlet fever; and they appear to contribute little to the control of infections such as influenza, pneumonia and the common cold.

These conclusions concerning the feasibility of control of infectious organisms according to their mode of spread require some modification in relation to developing countries, where the problems are much more difficult. This is partly because these countries cannot afford the costs of essential services; in 1970 it was estimated that only 14 per cent of their rural populations had ready access to safe drinking water and 8 per cent had adequate disposal of sewage. But it is also because climatic and geographical conditions in tropical and sub-tropical areas are particularly suitable for the propagation and transmission of many diseases which do not occur or are much less serious in the advanced countries. Some diseases of this type are water-borne (schistosomiasis and amoebic dysentery); many are animal-borne, the most important of them (malaria, yellow fever and trypanosomiasis) being transmitted by arthropod vectors. Hence the control of animal vectors is much more critical than in the developed world.

In summary, in technologically advanced countries it is relatively easy to control the transmission of water-borne infectious diseases; it is somewhat more difficult to control diseases spread by food, personal contact (particularly venereal infection) and animal vectors; and it is usually impossible to prevent transmission of airborne infections. In developing countries, because of limited resources it is difficult to provide safe water and efficient sewage disposal; and in tropical and sub-tropical areas, diseases spread by animal vectors are relatively more important than in temperate zones.

THE POST-REGISTRATION PERIOD

Airborne diseases
From the conclusion that it is usually impossible to prevent transmission of airborne infections, it would seem to follow that reduction of exposure to them has played little part in the fall of mortality. However, this conclusion needs some qualification.

Although it is difficult to prevent transmission of airborne diseases from one individual to another, less frequent exposure has nevertheless contributed to the decline of mortality from some infections. There are broadly two ways in which this has come about. The first is as a result of a reduction of the prevalence of a disease; smallpox, syphilis and tuberculosis are much less common than in the past, and exposure to them is correspondingly reduced. The second way is by improved living and working conditions, which prevent contact with infectious people in the community. It should be noted, however, that these influences are not equally effective with all airborne diseases. In the case of a highly infectious condition such as measles, in communities in which it is endemic nearly all children became infected, in spite of improvements in living conditions and a large reduction in the number of serious cases.

In several of the airborne infections associated with the decline of mortality (table 3.2) it is clear that prevention of exposure has contributed little if anything to the decrease in the number of deaths. The death rate from measles has fallen to a low level in technologically advanced countries; yet infection rates remain high. There is no effective control of the organisms which cause bronchitis and pneumonia, and the influences which determine the disappearance and reappearance of the influenza virus are not well understood. The streptococcus, which is responsible for scarlet fever and for most of the infections of the ear, pharynx and larynx, is ubiquitous, and the decline of these conditions owes little to reduced contact. However, in the case of the other diseases shown in table 3.2 – tuberculosis, whooping cough, diphtheria and smallpox – exposure to infection is undoubtedly less common than in the past, and I must now enquire whether this change has contributed substantially to the decline of mortality.

Although respiratory tuberculosis is not highly infectious, frequency and amount of exposure to the disease are undoubtedly important, and the only question is whether they have changed significantly. Infection occurred frequently at home or at work and was determined, not by general hygienic conditions such as water supply and sewage disposal, but by crowding. In the nineteenth century, new building of houses did little more than keep pace with the increase in the size of the population, and the number of persons per house in England and Wales fell only slightly (from 5·6 in 1801 to 5·3 in 1871). Exposure to infection at work must have increased during the first half of the nineteenth century, and it is unlikely that it was reduced substantially before its end. Newsholme, however, attached considerable importance to segregation of patients in sanatoria. While this may have been effective in the twentieth century, it can hardly have been so in the nineteenth, for by 1900 only a few sanatoria had been provided under voluntary auspices or by progressive local authorities, and most patients were still admitted to the Poor Law infirmaries. This is hardly surprising, since the tubercle bacillus was not identified until 1882.

In the twentieth century, however, exposure to tuberculosis has undoubtedly been reduced, partly by improved living and working conditions and use of sanatoria, but even more by the large reduction of the number of infectious patients in the community. In the nineteen fifties nearly all adolescents reacted positively to tuberculin (evidence that they had encountered the infection); today it is a minority which do so. It is therefore probable that although less frequent exposure may have contributed little to the decline of mortality from tuberculosis in the nineteenth century, it has been a significant influence in the twentieth. However, the reduction occurred mainly as a secondary consequence of the decline of morbidity and mortality brought about by other causes, rather than as a primary influence on the course of the disease.

The interpretation in the case of smallpox is in some respects similar. It is questionable whether any steps taken to reduce exposure to the infection have been effective. But other influences, particularly vaccination, have lowered mortality from smallpox, and eradication of the disease was undoubtedly assisted by the secondary effect of reduced contact.

Mortality from whooping cough declined from the seventh decade of the nineteenth century (figure 5.3). However, infection rates (indicated by the number of notifications) remained quite high, and fell rapidly only from about 1950. There is little reason to think that exposure to the disease was lowered much before this time, and it has occurred since as a result of a reduction in morbidity and mortality brought about by other influences.

Experience of diphtheria has been roughly parallel. Although case fatality fell from 1916–25, notifications remained high until 1940. The subsequent reduction of exposure indicated by the decline of notifications appears to have coincided with the introduction of immunization.

In summary, in some airborne infections (for example measles and scarlet fever) there are no grounds for thinking that even today the decline of mortality is due to reduced exposure. In others – tuberculosis, whooping cough, diphtheria and smallpox – there is little doubt that less frequent exposure has contributed to the fall of mortality. However, with the exception of smallpox and, possibly, tuberculosis, this influence was probably delayed until the twentieth century. Moreover it has come about, not as a primary influence, but as a secondary effect of other causes which reduced the prevalence of the diseases in the community.

Water- and food-borne diseases
What is known of the feasibility of control of the spread of infectious organisms indicates that it is in this class of diseases that a substantial reduction of mortality is likely to be achieved by prevention of exposure. The water- and food-borne diseases associated with the decline of the death rate since the mid-nineteenth century in England and Wales are shown in table 3.3. The table also includes typhus; since the disease

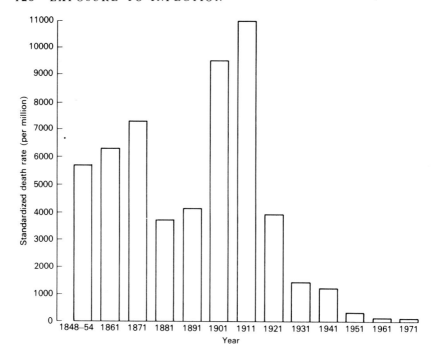

6.1 Diarrhoea and dysentery: death rates at ages 0–4, England and Wales.

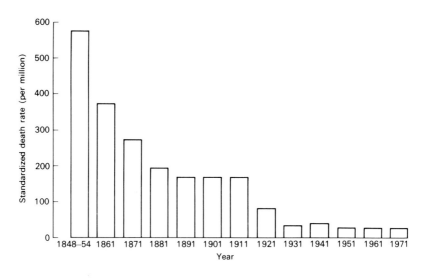

6.2 Diarrhoea and dysentery: death rates at ages 5 and over, England and Wales.

is vector-borne it is of course misplaced, but it was grouped with typhoid in national statistics before 1871.

The trend of the death rate from diarrhoeal diseases in table 3.3 is difficult to interpret, because there were cholera deaths in the period 1848–54 but none in 1901 and 1971. (The last epidemic was in 1865, so the reduction of the rate in part reflects the disappearance of cholera.) In assessing the decline of mortality from diarrhoeal diseases it is therefore preferable to exclude cholera deaths, and this treatment has been adopted in figures 6.1 and 6.2, which give death rates from diarrhoea and dysentery in persons aged 0–4, and 5 and over, respectively. The reason for distinguishing between these age groups is important. The deaths in infancy, particularly in the first year of life, were due largely to gastro-enteritis, which differs from the diseases associated with diarrhoea at later ages.

Figures 6.1 and 6.2 illustrate the significance of the distinction. For ages 5 and over, the death rate from diarrhoeal diseases declined from the mid-nineteenth century. At ages under 5, however, the rates were high in 1901 and 1911 (both had unusually warm summers) and it was only after 1911 that mortality fell continuously. This difference is attributable to the predominance of gastro-enteritis among causes of death in the first year of life.

As mentioned previously, because of inclusion of typhus deaths it is difficult to interpret the trend of mortality from enteric diseases before 1871. From that time, however, mean annual crude death rates for the next three decades were 320, 196 and 174. From 1901 the rates fell rapidly and (standardized) were in 1911, 83; 1921, 15; 1931, 6; 1941, 3; 1951, 0.

From the evidence it is clear that the death rate from water- and food-borne diseases declined continuously from the second half of the nineteenth century. (The exception is in respect of gastro-enteritis of infancy, where the decline of the death rate was delayed until the twentieth century.) Data from some other countries of Europe (Sweden, France and Ireland) are consistent with the same conclusion.[1]

There is no doubt that the fall of mortality from these diseases was due to reduced exposure brought about by improvements in hygiene. The trend owed nothing to immunization or therapy, and little if anything to a primary change in the character of the diseases. Their spread is due to defective sanitary arrangements, and their decline coincided with advances in hygiene, particularly, in the nineteenth century, purification of water and sewage disposal.

For many years the decline of gastro-enteritis presented a problem –

[1] T. McKeown, R. G. Brown and R. G. Record, 'An interpretation of the modern rise of population in Europe'. *Population Studies*, **20** (1972), p. 345.

a central one in the interpretation of infant mortality – which arose from uncertainty about the infective nature of the disease. Indeed in 1946, Topley and Wilson's classic text (*Principles of Bacteriology and Immunity*) divided enteritis of infancy into infective and non-infective types.[2] The division arose from failure to recognize that organisms which are usually harmless in adults and older children – particularly some strains of Escherichia coli – are often pathogenic in infancy. Hence it was not understood clearly that the higher mortality from gastroenteritis in artificially fed than in breast fed babies was due to the greater risk of contamination of artificial foods by micro-organisms. The control of gastro-enteritis, and the decline of infant mortality to which it contributed largely, required above all a safe milk supply.

The importance of milk in infancy was discussed recently by Beaver.[3] He attributed the reduction of infant mortality from 1900 mainly to improvements in the milk supply. Urban cow-keeping had almost died out by 1880, and milk was brought to towns by rail, which was more economical than the earlier practice of maintaining cattle in towns and transporting fodder in and manure out. However, the technical procedures required to make milk safe – cooling, heat treatment and bottling – were not available. In the present century commercial developments within the dairy industry favoured pathogen-free milk, in a fresh, condensed or dried form. Infant mortality, and particularly that due to gastro-enteritis, fell rapidly. This improvement coincided with the development of child welfare services, which emphasized the importance of safe infant feeding.

Taken with our present understanding of the infective origin of gastro-enteritis, this interpretation accounts in part for the high level of infant mortality in the late nineteenth century (when death rates were declining in older age groups), as well as for the rapid fall of the level from the beginning of this century. It also suggests an explanation for an observation which has sometimes puzzled historians, namely the relatively high mortality in well-to-do families in earlier centuries. It is probable that such families, although receiving sufficient food, were receiving infected food, and the contamination by micro-organisms was critical in early life. This point arises in the next chapter where it will be discussed more fully.

The other water- and food-borne disease which contributed substantially to the reduction of mortality was non-respiratory tuberculosis (table 3.3). The death rate from the disease declined from 1848–54; considerably in the second half of the nineteenth century and more rapidly after 1900 (figure 6.3). Although deaths due to human

[2] Topley and Wilson, *Principles of Bacteriology and Immunity*, revised by G. S. Wilson and A. A. Miles. Third edition, Arnold (London, 1946) pp. 1580–91.
[3] M. W. Beaver, 'Population, infant mortality and milk'. *Population Studies*, 27 (1973), p. 243.

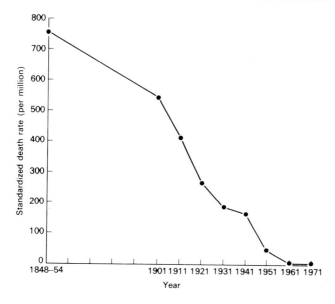

6.3 Non-respiratory tuberculosis: death rates, England and Wales.

and bovine infections cannot be separated in national statistics, it seems reasonable to believe that the human types were associated with the decline before 1900 and both types after 1900. In this case the explanation of the fall of mortality in the nineteenth century is in the same terms as for respiratory tuberculosis: it was not due to medical measures, or to a change in the character of the disease. (The main influence will be discussed in chapter 7.) The abdominal cases, however, were caused largely by infected milk, and their decline can be attributed to elimination of tuberculous cattle, and to the more general measures taken to protect milk supplies after 1900.

Other diseases due to micro-organisms
As noted earlier, most of the deaths shown under this heading were classified unsatisfactorily under convulsions and teething; several of them were undoubtedly due to airborne infections and their decline probably owed little to reduction of exposure. The infections (in table 3.4) which were affected were syphilis and puerperal fever, whose contributions to the decline of mortality were, however, very small. Moreover in the case of syphilis less frequent exposure was a result of another measure – treatment of the disease – which decreased the number of infective persons, rather than of a primary influence. In puerperal fever, exposure to infection was reduced by improved midwifery practice, following the teaching of Semmelweis.

THE EIGHTEENTH AND EARLY NINETEENTH CENTURIES

Since reliable information about the diseases which declined in the pre-registration period is not available, the contribution of less frequent exposure to infection must be assessed in general terms. It will be convenient to consider in turn airborne, water- and food-borne and vector-borne diseases.

In chapter 3 I concluded that there was probably a substantial reduction of mortality from airborne infections before 1838. It is unlikely that this was due substantially to less frequent exposure, since by increasing population size and the number of people in close contact, industrialization created optimum conditions for the propagation and spread of airborne infections, and this would have largely offset the reduction of exposure which might have been expected to result from their decreasing prevalence. Indeed the conditions which led to the predominance of infectious diseases, particularly of airborne type, following the first agricultural revolution ten thousand years earlier, were greatly extended in the nineteenth century. Many towns then had populations of the size required to maintain a disease such as measles, and the crowding of people at home and at work must have been ideal for the spread of tuberculosis.

In short, the trend of living conditions during the late eighteenth and early nineteenth centuries was such as to increase the risk of exposure to airborne infections and, if any reduction occurred, it could have come about only as a secondary consequence of other influences which diminished the incidence of disease. This possibility is illustrated by smallpox. As it became less prevalent, contact with it was reduced; but the change was a secondary rather than a primary influence.

However, it is in respect of water- and food-borne diseases that the question concerning exposure is most important. Here it is essential to distinguish clearly between measures of personal hygiene – washing, bathing, condition of clothing, etc. – which are within the control of the individual, and measures such as purification of water and disposal of sewage, whose effectiveness is determined by the quality of domestic and public services.

Standards of personal hygiene were low in the eighteenth century, particularly because bathing was uncommon, even among the well-to-do. They are believed to have improved by the mid-nineteenth century, but it is unlikely that this contributed significantly to the decline of mortality (except in the case of vector-borne disease referred to below). For it is the condition of the water and food which determines the risks of infection, rather than the cleanliness of the hands or utensils on which they are brought to the mouth. This point is illustrated by the observations that in a developed country, where hygienic standards are high, a young child is relatively safe, although his hands, mouth and clothing are frequently contaminated; whereas in a developing country, where hygiene is poor, scrupulous personal cleanliness alone is ineffective, and an individual must protect himself from infection by avoiding water unless it is boiled and by eating only cooked food.

It is upon purification of water, efficient disposal of sewage and food hygiene that reduction of exposure to water- and food-borne diseases primarily depends. There are good grounds for concluding that at least the first two of these influences deteriorated in the nineteenth century. In a vivid essay, Chapman described the circumstances which led to a crisis in London's sewage disposal system in the eighteen forties.

> The most apparent – and fundamental – precipitating factor was the increase in population. But Chadwick's zealous insistence on abolition of the cesspool was, paradoxically, an immediate precipitating factor. Prior to Chadwick's time, human excreta had been disposed of at or near the sites of their origin. Chadwick, by requiring the installation of flush toilets, moved the unwanted material well away from its myriad sites of origin, but gave insufficient thought to the effects of dumping such enormous quantities of sewage into the Thames in the London area. The result was the Great Stink, an infinitely more powerful stimulus to legislative action than Snow's work on transmission of cholera, or than the appallingly high death rates from the disease in the slum areas of east London, Southwark, Lambeth and Vauxhall.[4]

Although there may be some reservations about the last point, there should be none about the main conclusion: that the primitive sewage systems which served ineffectively in previous centuries, deteriorated under the pressures created by the greatly enlarged populations of the industrial towns. Their collapse carried its own risks and had unpleasant features to which Chapman refers; but, what was even more serious in relation to exposure to infectious disease, it led to further pollution of the sources on which the towns depended for their water. It was not until the second half of the nineteenth century that these risks were largely controlled – in London by new sewage systems and measures for purification of water supplies. But in the pre-registration period, and particularly its latter part, there is little doubt that exposure to water-borne diseases increased.

One can be less confident about the trend of food hygiene in the same period. What is clear is that there was little if any improvement in respect of milk, the most important component of the diet as a vehicle

---

[4] C. B. Chapman, 'The year of the Great Stink'. *Pharos* (July, 1972), p. 90.

for transmission of disease. In his examination of the relation between milk supplies, infant mortality and population growth, Beaver concluded that although the quantity of milk increased from the eighteenth century, it must often have been contaminated by pathogens.[5] It was not until the late nineteenth century that commercial pasteurization and bottling of milk began to be developed, and not until the twentieth century that a safe supply became generally available.

Since most solid foods are protected from contamination, not by sterilization and sealing as in the case of milk, but by precautions in handling and distribution involving many people, it is not possible to give a date in history when the transition from an infected to a safe supply was achieved. Indeed, as noted in the opening pages of this chapter, outbreaks of food poisoning still occur, even in advanced countries. However, it seems most unlikely that there was an improvement in food hygiene in the pre-registration period; on the contrary, it probably deteriorated, since the growth of towns made it necessary to transport large quantities of food from rural to urban areas, and thus resulted in increased handling and delayed consumption. A substantial advance in food hygiene was postponed until the present century, and rested largely on the work of microbiologists in the preceding fifty years.

To the conclusion that improvement in personal hygiene had little influence on the trend of mortality, an exception should possibly be made in the case of typhus. Unwashed bodies and infrequently changed clothing and bedding provide ideal conditions for the body lice which carry the organism, and the low standards of cleanliness which prevailed before the nineteenth century no doubt contributed, perhaps substantially, to the prevalence of typhus. Standards began to improve in the late eighteenth century, first among the well-to-do, but later in all classes, and this change may have had some effect on the fall of mortality. However, the epidemiology of the disease is complex, and it is unlikely that any single influence accounted for its decline and eventual disappearance.

To summarize: the feasibility of control of transmission of microorganisms is determined largely by the ways they are spread. It is relatively easy (in developed countries) to prevent exposure to waterborne diseases; it is more difficult to control those spread by food, personal contact and animal vectors; and it is usually impossible to prevent transmission of airborne infections.

There are no grounds for thinking that the reduction of mortality from airborne diseases such as measles and scarlet fever owes anything to reduced exposure. In others (tuberculosis, whooping cough,

---

[5] 'Population, infant mortality and milk', *op. cit.*

diphtheria and smallpox) less frequent contact contributed to the decline of the death rate; but this came about as a secondary consequence of other influences which lowered the prevalence of the diseases in the community.

The contribution of reduced exposure as a primary influence was mainly in control of water- and food-borne diseases. The improvement in water supplies and sewage disposal in the second half of the nineteenth century was largely responsible for the fall of mortality from enteric and diarrhoeal diseases at that time. The provision of a safe milk supply was the main reason for the reduction of deaths from gastro-enteritis and contributed substantially to the decline of infant mortality from 1900. The improvement in milk, together with elimination of tuberculous cattle also led to a decrease of the death rate associated with the bovine types of non-respiratory tuberculosis. In the eighteenth and nineteenth centuries, personal hygiene, particularly bathing, may have contributed to the decline of typhus.

In brief, as a primary influence, reduction of exposure to infection was important mainly in relation to diseases spread by water and food, and the basic measures were introduced progressively from the second half of the nineteenth century: purification of water; efficient disposal of sewage; provision of safe milk; and improved food hygiene. In the twentieth century these essentials were supported by advances in domestic, working and general environmental conditions. In other diseases (including some airborne infections such as tuberculosis and smallpox and a venereal infection in the case of syphilis), the trend of mortality was also influenced by reduced contact with infection as a secondary consequence of their diminished prevalence brought about by other measures.

7
Nutritional state

In the preceding chapters I concluded that the decline of mortality from infectious diseases was not due to a change in the character of the diseases, and that it owed little to reduced exposure to micro-organisms before the second half of the nineteenth century or to immunization and therapy before the twentieth. The possibility which remains is that the response to infection was modified by an advance in general health brought about by improvement in nutrition.

I recognize that this approach may suggest that I am seeking to prove by exclusion, on the principle enunciated by Sherlock Holmes: 'When we have eliminated the impossible, whatever remains, however improbable, must be the truth.' Certainly it is true that in deciding the order of the four chapters concerned with interpretation of the decline of the infectious diseases, I have had in mind my assessment of the relative importance of the different influences. But the reason for concluding that improvement in nutrition was the predominant influence on the fall of mortality in the eighteenth and nineteenth centuries is not essentially the negative one – that other explanations are inadequate. There are also positive grounds, which, since they are critical to the interpretation which follows, I must attempt at the outset to outline clearly.

In Britain there was a large increase in food supplies almost wholly, until the mid-nineteenth century, home produced. This increase made it possible to feed the expanded population without significant food imports; was it also the main reason for the growth of population? There were no clinical observations on individuals which enable us to conclude that there was a general improvement in nutrition between, say, 1700 and 1850; nor can it be shown conclusively that the food available per head of population increased. The evidence is indirect, but not on that account, less convincing. Extensive experience in developing countries leaves no doubt about the profound effect of nutritional state on response to micro-organisms; malnourished populations have higher infection rates and are more likely to die when infected. The predominance of infectious disease in pre- and early industrial societies was due largely to malnutrition, and an improvement in nutrition was a necessary condition for a substantial and prolonged reduction of mortality and growth of population. The fact that a large increase in food supplies coincided with a large increase of population therefore makes it reasonable to conclude that the one was the main reason for the other. This conclusion is derived essentially from present-day experience of infectious diseases, and is consistent with the findings that neither medical measures (immunization and therapy) nor reduction of exposure (at least as a primary influence) is likely to have had a substantial effect on the trend of mortality from the infections before the late nineteenth century.

The grounds for these conclusions will be discussed in the remainder of this chapter.

INCREASE IN FOOD SUPPLIES

Although price series of some agricultural products have been reconstructed from the late seventeenth century, estimates of food production were unreliable before the first agricultural census of Britain in 1865, and it was not until 1884 that national statistics of production and yield became available. The evidence that food production increased in the eighteenth and early nineteenth centuries is therefore of two kinds: circumstantial, from estimates of land areas under cultivation, yields per acre and amounts of imported and exported food; and inferential, from the fact that a greatly expanded population was fed on home grown food.

For what they are worth, estimates of grain and meat production in the eighteenth century suggest that it at least kept pace with the increasing population (in some years there was a small surplus of grain for export). However, during the last years of the century there was a succession of poor harvests, which led to widespread food shortages and forced the government to lift the ban on importation of animal products from Ireland and to prohibit exporting of grain. These difficulties were temporary, and during the first half of the nineteenth century both the amount of land devoted to cereal production and the yield per acre continued to increase. In 1840, the quantity of imported wheat relative to total consumption was no more than it had been in 1811 (about 5 per cent); but the population of Britain had increased during the interval by six and a half million (55 per cent). After 1885, imports of wheat, especially from North America, rose substantially and this permitted some reduction in the area of land used for wheat production in Britain. Imports of other foods also increased, and by 1870 about one fifth of the nation's food came from abroad.[1]

However I do not wish to place much emphasis on estimates of food production during the eighteenth and early nineteenth centuries. Evidence which is more convincing, and which I believe is not disputed, is that the greatly expanded population was fed on home grown food. The population of England and Wales increased from an estimated 5·5 million in 1702 to 8·9 in 1801 and 17·9 in 1851. Since exports and imports of food during this period were relatively small, it is clear that food production must have more than trebled to sustain an increase of 12·4 million in a century and a half.

Whether the population was better fed in the eighteenth and nineteenth centuries is another question and a central one in this context. Certainly there were no direct observations on the nutrition of individuals which would enable us to draw this conclusion; and from the conflicting views of economic historians about the trend of food production per head, it is clear that this type of evidence cannot decide whether nutrition improved during the period. I shall therefore approach the issue in quite a different way, by examining the relation between malnutrition and infectious disease in the later pages of this chapter.

ADVANCES IN AGRICULTURE

Although it is generally agreed that there was an increase in food production in the eighteenth and nineteenth centuries, there are differences of opinion about the nature of the advances in agriculture which led to it. From the second half of the nineteenth century the introduction of mechanization, chemical fertilizers and, later, insecticides, provide a sufficient explanation; but these methods were not available in the preceding century and a half when the initial large increase of food production occurred. Malthus, Ricardo and their contemporaries attributed the advance to extension of traditional methods (increased land use, manuring, winter feeding, rotation of crops, etc.), and this view was endorsed recently by Hutchinson, among others.[2] But it was not accepted by Langer in his review of 'American foods and Europe's population growth';[3] or by writers such as Arthur Young in the late eighteenth century and James Caird in the mid-nineteenth.

---

[1] T. McKeown, R. G. Brown and R. G. Record, 'An interpretation of the modern rise of population in Europe'. *Population Studies*, **26** (1972), p. 345.

[2] Sir Joseph Hutchinson, 'Land and human populations'. *The Advancement of Science*, **23** (1966), p. 241.

[3] W. L. Langer, 'American foods and Europe's population growth, 1750–1850'. *Journal of Social History*, Winter Number (1975), p. 51.

Langer attributed the increase in food essentially to the introduction of the potato and (in southern Europe) maize. However, since these crops were brought from the Americas in the sixteenth century, it seems permissible to regard their more intensive cultivation in the later period as part of the extension of traditional methods in which the explanation of the increased food production must presumably be sought.

A change from exploitive to productive agriculture (Hutchinson's terminology) occurred between 1650 and 1750 when British agriculture underwent major changes. The question whether they should be described as a technical revolution need not detain us. Fundamentally the changes comprised 'the establishment of the principle of the systemic conservation of fertility, by saving all manure, and distributing it uniformly over the land from which it was produced'.

The following developments were particularly important to the production and distribution of food.

(a) Organization. Enclosure, the major change in organization, began on a voluntary basis in the sixteenth century; it proceeded slowly in the seventeenth century but more rapidly in the eighteenth, so that it was well advanced by 1760 and almost complete by 1820. Even without improvements in technology, by encouraging more efficient farming, enclosure leads to increased productivity. But in Britain it also provided an essential basis for exploitation of the technological developments of the eighteenth and nineteenth centuries.

(b) Technology. Although there was some extension of the land under cultivation from the sixteenth to the eighteenth entury, the improvement in food supplies resulted mainly from increased productivity. Medieval agriculture had produced grain from arable fields and livestock from permanent grass lands with little attempt to balance crop and animal husbandry. The farming techniques introduced in the late seventeenth and early eighteenth centuries led to diversification and specialization. The predominant feature was the development of mixed farming, involving more intensive use of labour and spread more evenly over the seasons. The following were among the important developments:

(i) New crops. These included clover and other leguminous hays in use in the Low Countries in the seventeenth century and, particularly, root crops. The term root crops covers two categories (a) tap roots (e.g. turnips, beets, carrots and parsnips) which propagate only by seed and (b) tubers (e.g. the yams and casava of the tropics) which propagate vegetatively. All the native root crops of the temperate zone of the Old World are of the tap root type; they were introduced to Britain, probably from the Low Countries, in the seventeenth century. Of the tubers, only the potato and the Jerusalem artichoke have been brought from America into the cooler regions of the Old World.[4] In some parts of Europe the potato was important in the sixteenth and seventeenth centuries, but it was grown extensively in England for human consumption only from about 1750 although it may have been used a little earlier for fodder.

In his full discussion of 'American foods and Europe's population growth', Langer concluded that 'the sudden growth of the European population was due in large measure to a substantial increase in the food supply', and that the significant advance in agriculture was extensive cultivation of the potato and maize.[5] Certainly there seems little doubt that the potato was the predominant influence on the growth of population in Ireland, a conclusion which is strongly suggested by the disastrous consequence of the crop failures in the nineteenth century. We should also note in passing that the high mortality – more than a million people died – was due largely to infectious diseases such as diarrhoea and typhus associated with malnutrition, rather than to overt starvation.

Whether the potato (and maize in the south) had quite the same predominance in other parts of Europe is another question; certainly England and Wales were never so dependent as Ireland on the single crop. Even so, it is quite possible that the potato, with its enormous return in calories for a unit of land, made a much more significant contribution to the increase in food supplies in the eighteenth and nineteenth centuries than that which has been recognized hitherto.

(ii) Crop rotation, which broke the pattern of traditional grain-fallow rotation, has been traced from the middle Rhine valley in the sixteenth century, through the Low Countries to England at some time in the seventeenth. Different rotations were practised in different parts of the country but the principles were the same.

(iii) Conservation of fertility. Hutchinson considered this the most important of all the developments.[6] Marling of light soils and liming of heavy soils were practised in the seventeenth century and agricultural use of urban waste products is likely to have increased with increasing population density. But the most significant contribution to fertility conservation was probably the development of mixed farming, based on new crops, new

---

[4] L. Hogben, personal communication.
[5] 'American foods and Europe's population growth', op. cit.
[6] 'Land and human populations', op. cit.

rotations and enclosure, leading to a better balance between animal and plant husbandry. Although early in the eighteenth century Tull recognized the importance of Glauber's discovery (about 1650) that saltpetre renews exhausted soils, chemical fertilizers were not used widely until the second half of the nineteenth century.[7]

(iv) Seed production. In Elizabethan times, farmers relied on dredge corn and hayloft sweepings to seed cereals. There are references to commercial seed production as early as 1652, but the use of seed, for example in production of turnips and clover, developed very slowly.[7]

(v) Winter feeding. The increased supplies of clover and root crops made it possible to provide winter food for animals which formerly would have had to be killed. During the eighteenth century this led to a large increase in meat production. However, there was little selective breeding before 1750, and it seems likely that the increase in carcass weight during the eighteenth century was exaggerated by some writers.

(vi) Farm implements. Although there were some improvements in traditional implements, the only major change during the eighteenth century was the introduction of the smaller, lighter, triangular plough with curved mould board, which could be pulled by fewer beasts and worked by one man. However, Hogben also attached importance to the mechanical drill, invented by Tull in 1701, although not in general use until considerably later.[7] The drill made it possible to prevent wind waste of seeds which had restricted progress in crop production.

(c) Transport. There were improvements in coastal navigation, in navigable rivers and in roads during the seventeenth and eighteenth centuries, but the most significant change prior to the construction of railways in the nineteenth century was the development of canals from the middle of the eighteenth. These improvements were essential to the distribution of food, particularly since areas of production were unevenly distributed throughout the country.

In concluding this brief account of developments in British agriculture, two other points should be mentioned. Although many of the changes which led to the increase in food production in the eighteenth century coincided more or less with early industrialization, the nature of the changes (they were neither chemical nor mechanical) suggests that technically at least they were independent of it. The other point is that many of the advances in agriculture in Britain were in widespread use at the same period or earlier, elsewhere in Europe.

[7] Hogben, *op. cit.*

MALNUTRITION AND INFECTIOUS DISEASE

It is well recognized that the state of health of an individual has a profound bearing on his reaction to infectious disease. Measles is a conspicuous example of a condition in which infection rates are high in all social classes, but the likelihood of serious illness and death depends largely on the health of the child and is much increased among the poor. It is also clear that the general state of health is determined by multiple influences, including particularly previous illnesses and nutrition.

It is more difficult to go beyond these generalizations to a precise estimate of the part played by nutrition in determining the outcome of an infectious disease. There are many conflicting reports in the literature, and disorders of metabolism and deficiency diseases were accorded a relatively minor role in the health of man and animals until recently. However, Newberne and Williams have reviewed the effects of nutritional influences on the course of infections. 'The ultimate effect of an infection depends to a considerable degree on the nutritional adequacy of the animal at the time of exposure to the agent. A severe degree of deficiency of almost any of the essential nutrients may have a marked effect on the manner in which the host responds to the effect of an infectious agent. Abundant evidence clearly indicates that the same infection may be mild or even inapparent in a well nourished animal, but virulent and sometimes fatal in one that is malnourished.' They refer to four ways in which nutrition influences infection: '1) effects on the host which facilitate initial invasion of the infectious agent; 2) through an effect on the agent once it is established in the tissues; 3) through an effect on secondary infection; or 4) by retarding convalescence after infection.' They conclude that: 'Grossly inadequate intakes of protein and other specific nutrients are today resulting in extreme degrees of malnutrition and concomitant infectious disease. It seems likely that the interaction between nutrition and infection are more important in animal and human populations than one would predict from the results of laboratory investigations. It must be remembered that the interaction between nutrition and infection is dynamic, being frequently characterized by synergism and less commonly, by antagonism, and that control of malnutrition and infection are interdependent, so that the course of a disease is intimately related to the nutritional status of the host.'

In man also, although the relationship is not in doubt, it has proved difficult to obtain unequivocal results, for as food shortage and

[8] P. M. Newberne and G. Williams, 'Nutritional influences on the course of infections'. In *Resistance to Infectious Disease*, edited by R. H. Dunlop and H. W. Moon, Saskatoon Modern Press (1970), p. 93.

other features of poverty usually occur together, their respective contributions to mortality are hard to separate. For example, populations in which tuberculosis, or in a tropical country, schistosomiasis, are common are likely to be poor, underfed and exposed to infection; and it is not easy to determine the relative importance of malnutrition and frequent exposure. There is some evidence of a quasi-experimental kind in the increased incidence of infectious diseases in populations whose food intake was reduced substantially during the two world wars.

However, knowledge of the relation between malnutrition and infection has been extended considerably in recent years through experience acquired by the World Health Organization in developing countries, where infectious diseases are still predominant. This experience leaves no doubt that malnutrition contributes largely to the high level of infectious deaths; the populations are more prone to infections and suffer more seriously when they are infected. Moreover, infectious diseases have an unfavourable effect on nutritional state, and the interaction between disease and malnutrition leads to a vicious cycle which is characteristic of poverty and underdevelopment. These effects are not restricted to respiratory and intestinal infections for which there are no specific vaccines; mortality is still high from measles and whooping cough for which effective immunization is available, and indeed it is questionable whether infectious diseases can be controlled by vaccination in a malnourished population. The problems are particularly serious in infancy, before the child has developed its own natural defence mechanisms. The World Health Organization concluded that 'one half to three quarters of all statistically recorded deaths of infants and young children are attributed to a combination of malnutrition and infection.'[9] The deficiency is due mainly to lack of calories and proteins, although mineral and vitamin deficiencies are frequently associated.

It should be emphasized that the malnutrition which is the common background of infectious diseases in developing countries is not necessarily, and it is not usually of the overt types such as rickets, beriberi, pellagra and the protein-calorie deficiency syndromes, kwashiokor and marasmus; it is more often manifested as chronic malnutrition without specific features which are easily recognized. Two thirds of the populations of some countries are estimated to suffer from this less obvious kind of deficiency, in which infection is frequently the final influence which results in death. The interpretation of this experience was discussed in a recent report from the World Health Organization.

[9] World Health Organization, 'Better food for a healthier world'. *Features* FS/19 (1973).

A debilitated organism is far less resistant to attacks by invading micro-organisms. Ordinary measles or diarrhoea – harmless and short-lived diseases among well fed children – are usually serious and often fatal to the chronically malnourished. Before vaccines existed, practically every child in all countries caught measles, but 300 times more deaths occurred in the poorer countries than in the richer ones. The reason was not that the virus was more virulent, nor that there were fewer medical services; but that in poorly nourished communities the microbes attack a host which, because of chronic malnutrition, is less able to resist. The same happens with diarrhoea, respiratory infections, tuberculosis and many other common infections to which malnourished populations pay a heavy and unnecessary toll.[12]

The same report gave the results of a recent investigation of mortality in infancy in Latin America, which concluded that 'when malnutrition was not given as the major cause of death in official statistics, it was an associated cause in 57 per cent of all deaths among children under five and, in some regions, in two thirds of these deaths. Diarrhoeal infections accounted for most of the deaths, with malnutrition as an associated cause in 50–80 per cent of cases. Malnutrition was also a concomitant factor in 60 per cent of the deaths attributable to measles.'[12] The author concluded that malnutrition was the most serious health problem among the populations studied.

These and other investigations show the enormous importance of nutrition in determining the outcome of infection, and the tragic synergistic relation which exists between malnutrition and infectious disease. The World Health Organization report suggests that 'we have given too much attention to the enemy and have to some extent overlooked our own defences.'[10] That is to say we have concentrated on specific measures such as vaccination and environmental improvement without sufficient regard for the predominant part played by nutritional state. 'For the time being,' it concluded, 'an adequate diet is the most effective "vaccine" against most of the diarrhoeal, respiratory and other common infections.'

INFECTIOUS DISEASES AFTER THE FIRST AGRICULTURAL REVOLUTION

It is against the background of this present-day understanding of the relation between malnutrition and infectious disease that experience of the infections in the period before their decline must be interpreted. The conclusion that the beginning of the modern rise of

[10] M. Behar, 'A deadly combination'. *World Health* (February–March, 1974), p. 29.

population resulted from an increase in food supplies rests largely on the belief that the size of human populations had been limited previously by lack of food, and that an increase was a necessary condition for a substantial and prolonged expansion. I must now examine the grounds for this viewpoint.

Until about 10,000 years ago, the main restraint on population growth was a high level of mortality determined directly or indirectly by lack of food. (This conclusion was discussed in chapter 3.) The increase in food supplies which resulted from the first agricultural revolution lowered mortality and led to an expansion of numbers, an expansion which continued to the point at which food resources became again marginal. This is of course no more than a restatement of the Malthusian interpretation, which can, however, be extended in the light of knowledge of the infections. The aggregation of populations of substantial size created the conditions required for the propagation and transmission of micro-organisms, particularly those that are airborne. Many organisms did not survive contact with man; others achieved a relationship which was unharmful and, occasionally, mutually beneficial; a minority caused sickness and death of heir hosts. However, the effects of this minority of micro-organisms on human health were so devastating that infectious diseases became the predominant cause of death, something they had not been during man's evolution and are not today for other animals living in their natural habitats.

But although this may describe the circumstances under which infectious diseases became predominant, it does not account for the significance of malnutrition; indeed at first sight it would appear to be an advantage for a parasite to have a well fed host, and surprising that an improvement in human nutrition since the eighteenth century should have been a disaster for certain micro-organisms.

For most micro-organisms it is probably desirable to have a well nourished host, and no disadvantages have resulted to them from the better nutrition of the past few centuries. But the relationship between man and organisms which cause disease is unstable, and finely balanced according to the physiological state of host and parasite. It was critical to this relationship that it evolved over a period when the human host was, in general, poorly nourished, because numbers had expanded beyond the point at which they could be maintained in health by the available food resources. It is therefore understandable that an improvement in human health, brought about by an advance in nutrition, should have tipped the balance of advantage in favour of the host and against the parasite. Hence the better nutrition was a necessary condition for a substantial and prolonged decline of mortality; without it immunization and therapy would have been of little value and reduction of exposure to some organisms less effective. This theoretical appraisal of the relation between malnutrition and infection is entirely in keeping with extensive recent experience in developing countries, described above.

It is unfortunate that the infections which declined cannot be identified reliably before 1838. They no doubt included typhus and smallpox, but it is unlikely that these diseases were sufficiently common to account for a substantial proportion of the total reduction of mortality. In the years after registration tuberculosis was the predominant cause of death, and since the death rate from the disease was declining rapidly from the time of registration, it seems probable that it was doing so at least in the years immediately before. Whether tuberculosis had the same importance in the eighteenth century is another question.

However, present-day experience in developing countries again suggests what may be offered, with reservations, as a possible answer. There is little doubt that the reduction of mortality in the eighteenth and early nineteenth centuries occurred predominantly in childhood. The improvement in nutrition would have lowered the number of deaths from all or nearly all the common infections, including the respiratory and, particularly, the diarrhoeal diseases. Indeed the investigations in Latin America referred to above suggest that the diarrhoeal diseases, which accounted for most of the deaths in childhood, are likely to have been those chiefly affected.

This interpretation is consistent with evidence from national statistics for England and Wales (after 1838), although it leaves open the question of the relative importance of tuberculosis before and after registration. It is also uncertain whether the improvement in childhood mortality affected children in the first year of life. The fact that infant mortality was 150 (per thousand live births) when first recorded in 1838, suggests that the rate may have fallen earlier; and Beaver suggested that 'a reduction in this rate was associated with agricultural and commercial developments during the second half of the eighteenth century, whereby cow's milk was made generally available both in town and country throughout the year.'[11] He also concluded that 'a further reduction in infant mortality took place at the beginning of this century; this was associated with commercial development within the dairy industry which favoured a pathogen-free milk.' That is to say the first major advance in infancy resulted from an increase in the amount of milk, and the second from an improvement in its safety.

This conclusion in respect of the first year of life is broadly in accord with the interpretation suggested for the decline of mortality at later ages (but still predominantly in childhood). The death rate fell in the eighteenth and nineteenth centuries because of an increase in food

[11] M. W. Beaver, 'Population, infant mortality and milk'. *Population Studies*, **27** (1973), p. 243.

supplies which led to better nutrition. From the second half of the nineteenth century this advance was strongly supported by reduction of exposure to infection which resulted indirectly from the falling prevalence of disease, and directly from improved hygiene affecting, in the first instance, the quality of water and food.

FOOD, INFECTION AND THE ARISTOCRACY

I should now consider a possible objection to the conclusion that an increase in food supplies was the predominant influence on the growth of population in the eighteenth and nineteenth centuries. It is that the expectation of life of well-to-do people appears to have increased over the same period, although they presumably had sufficient food and hence. would not be expected to provide scope for a substantial improvement in nutrition.[12]

The evidence concerning the well-to-do in Britain is based on a study of the dates of birth and death of British peers born in the sixteenth, seventeenth and eighteenth centuries.[13] The data improved during this period and those for the final cohort (1775–99) are reasonably accurate. However, the earlier observations are less reliable and for the 1700–24 cohort only 70 per cent of the birth dates were known within a few years. Errors of this order could have a considerable influence on estimates of life expectation.

There are also some difficulties of interpretation. For example, the patterns observed for males and females are rather different, so that the sexes must be considered separately. For males, there were large increases in life expectancy at birth for the second and third cohorts of the eighteenth century, but the substantial improvement of the third cohort over the second was reduced by the age of five and still further by the age of 15. This suggests that the major contribution to improved life expectation at birth for the 1750–74 cohort was a decline in child, and particularly infant mortality, and this is supported by more direct measures of mortality. On the other hand, the 1725–49 birth cohort continued to show improvement up to the age of 65, over and above that of surrounding cohorts (the preceding one in particular, which was most fully 'exposed' to the eighteenth century, showed very little improvement from the age of 35, i.e. from 1735–60). For males aged over 55, however, there was little change in life expectancy during the eighteenth century until about 1780.

For females, the major improvement at birth was concentrated

[12] P. E. Razzell, 'An interpretation of the modern rise of population in Europe – a critique'. *Population Studies*, **28** (1974), p. 1.

[13] T. H. Hollingsworth, 'The demography of the British peerage'. *Supplement to Population Studies*, **18** (1964), p. 57.

within the 1750–74 birth cohort; it was almost halved by age 5 (again indicating a substantial fall in infant mortality), though still considerable (5½ years over the previous cohort). Otherwise, at all ages from 25 to 55, and for all cohorts living through the eighteenth century from the 1675–99 birth cohort to that of 1750–74, there seems to have been a more or less uniform increase in life expectation between each cohort and the next. This is not seen in earlier cohorts (those aged 25 and over in 1700).

With due regard for some deficiencies of this evidence, it suggests that there was a substantial increase in expectation of life of the British aristocracy, at least from the mid-eighteenth century, due mainly to reduction of mortality in early life.

How is this advance to be explained if it cannot, as I agree, be attributed plausibly to improvement in nutrition? A possible approach to this question is to consider in turn the other influences which lowered mortality in the general population at a later date, and enquire whether they might have had an earlier effect on the health of the aristocracy.

With the exception of vaccination against smallpox, the contribution of immunization and therapy was delayed until the twentieth century. Since the delay was due to lack of knowledge, there is no reason to think that these influences were effective earlier in the case of well-to-do people.

Purification of water and efficient disposal of sewage depend mainly on public measures, and the aristocracy are unlikely to have benefited much in advance of the population as a whole (in the second half of the nineteenth century). Conceivably they had some advantage from better personal hygiene, for example the earlier use of water closets, and more frequent bathing and cleaner bedding which might have affected experience of typhus. The condition of their food might also have improved somewhat earlier, although probably not in the case of milk, the single most important component of the diet in childhood, for which the means of pasteurization, bottling and distribution were not available before 1900. Indeed, as noted in the preceding chapter, it is likely that well-to-do families, while having sufficient food, were eating infected food, and this alone would account for a high death rate in early childhood. The frequent references in Dorothy Wordsworth's journal to her own and William's troubles with their bowels are an indication that food hygiene in Dove Cottage, as no doubt in the homes of the upper and middle classes in general, left a good deal to be desired.

But even if these relatively minor advances in personal hygiene occurred, they seem insufficient to explain a substantial reduction of mortality in aristocratic families, and for a possible explanation we must consider more closely the question of exposure to infection. In respect of the population as a whole the interpretation suggested for the decline of deaths from infectious diseases before the twentieth century is as follows: initially it was due to improvement in general health brought about by better nutrition; from the second half of the nineteenth century hygienic measures in respect of water, sewage and food (particularly milk) reduced exposure to infection. But it should also be recognized that quite apart from these specific measures, the lower prevalence of infectious diseases which resulted from improved nutrition must have diminished the frequency of exposure, in this case however as a secondary rather than a primary influence. For the majority of people, the advantages of lower prevalence would no doubt have been offset in the nineteenth century by deteriorating working and living conditions which brought large numbers into close contact and led to a decline in hygienic standards, particularly in respect of water and sewage disposal. But the aristocracy would have avoided these penalties of industrialization, while benefiting from the lower prevalence of many micro-organisms. It should be noted that this conclusion turns on a secondary effect (reduced exposure) in well-to-do people, of a primary influence (better nutrition) in the general population.

That this is not merely a theoretical possibility can be illustrated from experience of tuberculosis in the nineteenth and early twentieth centuries. The disease occurred in wealthy people, although less frequently and less seriously than among the poor. The difference between the social classes was determined partly by different frequencies of exposure, but also by the better nutrition of the well-to-do, which reduced both the likelihood and the severity of the illness. Nevertheless, mortality from tuberculosis undoubtedly declined in the middle and upper classes, as in the population as a whole, long before the introduction of effective treatment in 1947. It declined because the disease had become less prevalent in the community as a result of a general improvement in nutrition. Thus well-to-do people benefited from a secondary effect of improved nutrition, for which they themselves offered little scope.

This experience of tuberculosis since registration suggests the direction in which we should look for the explanation of the increased expectation of life of the aristocracy in the eighteenth century. In chapter 3 I concluded that mortality from infectious diseases declined in the period before registration of births, as it undoubtedly declined subsequently. This trend I attribute mainly to an advance in nutrition, supported by vaccination against smallpox and, possibly, in the case of typhus, by better personal hygiene. As a result of the falling prevalence of the diseases, exposure to them must also have diminished, and in different degrees this would have contributed to the health of all social classes. In the nineteenth century this advantage would have been offset to some extent for most people (but not for the aristocracy) by the effects of conditions in the industrial towns.

To summarize: from the time of the first agricultural revolution (about 10,000 years ago) infectious diseases were the predominant cause of death. The relationship between man and micro-organisms which cause disease evolved over a period when the human host was, in general, poorly nourished, and an improvement in nutrition was a necessary condition for a substantial and prolonged decline of mortality. This conclusion is in keeping with extensive recent experience in developing countries, which leaves no doubt that malnourished populations are more prone to infections and suffer more seriously when they are infected. The malnutrition which is the common background of infectious diseases is not usually of the overt types such as rickets, beri-beri, pellagra and the protein calorie deficiency syndromes, kwashiokor and marasmus; it is more often manifested as chronic malnutrition without specific features which are easily recognized.

In Europe there was a large increase in food supplies between the end of the seventeenth century and the mid-nineteenth, in Britain sufficient to feed a population that had trebled in size, without significant imported food. This increase coincided with a substantial reduction of mortality from infectious diseases and, it is suggested, was the main reason for it. The decrease of deaths was predominantly in childhood and, less certainly, in infancy; it probably affected all, or nearly all the common infections, including the respiratory and, particularly, the diarrhoeal diseases. What is uncertain is whether tuberculosis had the predominant place among the causes of death which declined in the eighteenth century which it undoubtedly had in the nineteenth. From the second half of the nineteenth century the improvement in health which resulted from the advance in nutrition was supported powerfully by a reduction of exposure to infection, brought about indirectly by the falling prevalence of disease, and directly by improved hygiene affecting, in the first instance, the quality of water and food.

8
Non-infective conditions

In the preceding four chapters, I discussed reasons for the decline of mortality from infectious diseases. In England and Wales they were associated with about three quarters of the decrease of the death rate between the time of registration and the present day; indeed with the exceptions of infanticide and starvation, about which information is understandably incomplete, it is unlikely that any non-infective conditions contributed substantially to the improvement in health before the twentieth century. From 1900, however, the reduction of deaths from non-infective conditions was considerable, and to complete the interpretation of the fall of mortality in the past three centuries, it is necessary to account for it. From 1838 this can be done by examining the causes of death which declined, but in the eighteenth and early nineteenth centuries one must again rely on a more general appraisal.

THE POST-REGISTRATION PERIOD

It was shown in table 3.5 that about a quarter (25·6 per cent) of the total decline of mortality between 1848–54 and 1971 was associated with conditions not attributable to micro-organisms. Approximately a tenth of this reduction (10 per cent of 25·6 per cent) occurred before 1901.

In chapter 3, the trend in deaths from non-infective conditions in the nineteenth century was attributed mainly to errors in certification of cause of death; it was suggested that as the standard of diagnosis gradually improved, deaths were assigned to other and, in general, more accurate causes. This probably explains the substantial fall between 1848–54 and 1901 in death rates from 'old age' and 'other diseases', which together accounted for about four fifths of the decline of mortality from non-infective conditions. It was concluded that the Registrar General's statistics provide no convincing evidence of a decrease of non-infective causes of death before 1901. A reservation concerning the possible significance of infanticide and starvation, neither of which is represented fully in the Registrar General's classification, is referred to below. With this exception, the problem of interpreting the reduction of mortality from non-infective conditions arises in the present century.

As noted in chapter 3, the effect of the decline of non-infective conditions on the total decrease of the death rate was offset to a considerable extent by the increase in mortality due to lung cancer and myocardial infarction, brought about by smoking and other influences. In the brief discussion which follows of reasons for the decline of deaths from non-infective conditions in this century, the effect of these increases will be ignored, and the causes of death associated with the decline will be referred to in order according to their contribution to the reduction of the death rate.

Much the largest fall (1057 deaths per million between 1901 and 1971) was associated with the heterogeneous class, 'prematurity, immaturity and other diseases of infancy' (table 3.5). These deaths were almost restricted to the first year of life, and their contribution to the decline of infant mortality was of the same order of magnitude as that of deaths due to gastroenteritis. In 1901 more than 90 per cent of them were certified under two headings, 'premature birth' and 'atrophy, debility'. The latter no longer appears in the Registrar General's classification, so that the large decrease in the number of deaths is explained by transfers to other causes of death (many of which have of course declined). 'Premature birth' had no consistent meaning in 1901; it was later identified with low birth weight until the internationally agreed basis was changed, to take account of the duration of gestation. With due regard for these inconsistencies, there has undoubtedly been a large reduction in deaths of this type in the first year of life. This contribution to the decline of the non-infective death rate was probably due in part to a rising standard of living – particularly improvement in maternal nutrition which lowered the incidence of premature birth – and in part to improved obstetric care (before and during labour) and better management of the premature infant.

Nothing further need be said about deaths attributed to 'old age' in 1901, whose rapid decline was evidently due to transfers to more satisfactory diagnoses. Next in magnitude (according to their contribution to the fall of the death rate) were 'other diseases', which comprised a considerable number of causes of death, many of which would today be unacceptable. The largest reductions were associated with alcoholism, rickets and non-infective diseases of the respiratory system other than emphysema and asthma, and are probably explained in part by less frequent drinking, improved nutrition and, particularly in the case of the respiratory diseases, by better certification. There were also some causes of death (for example eczema) whose decline was no doubt largely due to treatment.

'Other diseases of digestive system' exclude cancers, but include some causes of death whose decrease was due to better classification (for example, gastric catarrh). The largest reductions appear to have been associated with diseases now treated by surgery (gall bladder disease, hernia and intestinal obstruction) and with cirrhosis whose decline is attributable to less frequent drinking.

The next two classes – rheumatic heart disease and nephritis – are essentially infective and are misplaced in this discussion. They have been included only because (as noted in chapter 3) table 3.5 examined the trend of mortality in the nineteenth as well as the twentieth century, and for 1848–54 these infections cannot be separated from non-infective causes of death. To this extent the estimate of the contribution of non-infective conditions to the fall of the death rate is overstated.

There seems little doubt that the decline of mortality from violence in the twentieth century, when the frequency of accidents has risen steadily, was due predominantly to surgery.

The deaths under 'other diseases of nervous system' include brain tumour, diseases of the cord and neuritis where diagnoses must be in doubt. The improvement was mainly in respect of epilepsy, and may be attributed to treatment. The reasons for the reduction of the death rate from cerebro-vascular disease is not clear, and the contributions of the two remaining classes (other diseases of urinary system and pregnancy and childbirth – excluding sepsis) were small.

From this analysis it is evident that interpretation of the trend of non-infective causes of death can be attempted only in very general terms; the influences are more varied and less specific than in the case of the infections. Therapeutic measures made a substantial contribution in respect of some causes of death; for example there is little doubt about the value of surgery in cases of violence and in several digestive conditions. It is not possible to be equally confident about the effects of treatment on some other conditions listed in table 3.5. The heterogeneous class of deaths ascribed to 'prematurity, immaturity, other diseases of infancy' made the largest contribution to the total decline of mortality. These deaths were almost restricted to the first year of life, and their reduction, together with that of deaths due to gastroenteritis, was the main reason for the rapid fall of infant mortality from the beginning of this century. While this trend no doubt owed something to improvements in obstetric services, before and during labour, it was probably due mainly to advances in maternal nutrition and better infant feeding and care. Some of the decline shown in table 3.5 was associated with changes in classification of causes of death, and in two cases at least (rheumatic fever and nephritis) was due to inclusion of what were essentially infectious causes of death.

THE EIGHTEENTH AND EARLY NINETEENTH CENTURIES

Since causes of death cannot be identified in the pre-registration period, one must rely (as in chapter 5) on an examination of developments in the eighteenth century which might have led to a reduction of mortality from non-infective conditions. They include advances in surgery and medicine, and the provision of hospital and dispensary services. In addition, however, there is the important question whether the decline of infanticide and starvation contributed substantially to the fall of the death rate. Since I have come to believe that this is perhaps the most important issue related to non-infectious deaths in the pre-registration period, it will be convenient to consider it first.

Infanticide

In chapter 3 I referred to Langer's review of the history of infanticide, which suggested that it was practised on a substantial scale, at least until the second half of the nineteenth century, and probably in some developing countries until the present day.[1] Although this conclusion cannot be supported by statistics – for obvious reasons infanticide is not reported fully in national classifications of cause of death – it is nevertheless consistent with extensive historical evidence assembled by Langer and many others. An indication is the fact that Stevenson and his family were surprised to find that there were few children in the populations they encountered in the islands of the Pacific; there is little doubt about the explanation.

But although infanticide was probably common in the eighteenth and previous centuries, it is not possible to judge with any precision when the practice declined. However, it seems likely that it became somewhat less frequent as the growth of foundling hospitals made it possible for a mother to transfer an unwanted child rather than destroy it. This development is well illustrated by the experience of a foundling hospital in St Petersburg, described by Langer: 'By the mid 1830s it had 25,000 children on its rolls and was admitting 5000 newcomers annually. Since no questions were asked and the place was attractive, almost half of the newborn babies were deposited there by their parents. A dozen doctors and 600 wet-nurses were in attendance to care for the children during the first six weeks, after which they were sent to peasant nurses in the country. At the age of six (if they survived to that age) they were

[1] W. L. Langer, 'Infanticide: a historical survey'. *History of Childhood Quarterly*, **I** (1974), p. 353.

returned to St Petersburg for systematic education. The programme was excellent, but its aims were impossible to achieve. Despite all excellent management and professional efforts, thirty to forty per cent of the children died during the first six weeks and hardly a third reached the age of six.'[2] In England, Parliament (in 1756) made provision for asylums for exposed or deserted young children to be opened in all counties, ridings and divisions of the kingdom; and in France, Napoleon decreed (in 1811) that there should be hospitals in every department. However, the demand was far beyond the resources of the foundling institutions, and it was not until the last quarter of the nineteenth century that the practice of infanticide became uncommon and not until the twentieth that (in western Europe) it virtually disappeared. Its decline occurred over approximately the same period as the fall of the birth rate, and while many other developments may have contributed (for example improved living conditions and maternal and child welfare services) the main influence was undoubtedly the growth of contraceptive practices which reduced the number of unwanted births.

Starvation

This is the other important non-infective cause of death which may have declined significantly in the pre-registration period and later. Again, statistical evidence is deficient. Moreover, as noted in chapter 7, unless food supplies are grossly deficient, there are many more cases of chronic malnutrition, frequently associated with infectious diseases but without definitive signs, than there are cases with specific evidence (such as rickets or kwashiokor) of deficiency or frank starvation. But if the general conclusion is accepted – that the nutrition of the population was poor at the beginning of the eighteenth century and has improved continuously since that time – it seems inevitable that some people must have been at or near starvation level and that their number decreased. This conclusion is not difficult to accept for the eighteenth and nineteenth centuries, when it is recognized that even in the most advanced and wealthiest countries there are sections of the population who are underfed even in the present day.

Surgery

There is little difficulty in coming to a conclusion about eighteenth-century surgery. Before the introduction of anaesthesia, operations were almost restricted to the following: amputation, lithotomy, trephining of the skull, incision of abscess and operation for cataract. For a modern reader, the circumstances in which these procedures were carried out are almost unbelievable. The discovery of the anaesthetic properties of

[2] *Ibid.*

nitrous oxide in 1800, and a practical demonstration of the use of ether in 1846, greatly extended the scope of surgery. It did not increase its safety, and as recently as the last quarter of the nineteenth century results of the common operations were, by any standards, appalling. In 1874 the senior surgeon to University College Hospital reviewed thirty years' experience with surgery, and concluded that 'skill in the performance has far outstripped the success in the result.'[3] He showed that mortality following all forms of amputation was between 35 and 50 per cent, and following certain forms it was as high as 90 per cent. These figures were based on the work of the most expert surgeons, working in the largest hospitals, and are probably no worse than would have been obtained elsewhere; indeed in continental hospitals at the same period mortality was even higher. Results of other types of operation were equally bad; it was not until the introduction of anti-septic procedures that surgery became relatively safe. Ericksen's observations were based upon the third quarter of the nineteenth century; there is certainly no reason to suppose that earlier results were better, and Singer was unquestionably correct in his judgement that 'surgery had an almost inappreciable effect on vital statistics, until the advent of Anaesthesia and Antiseptics.'[4] Indeed, from the point of view of the surgeon this is a generous judgement.

Medicines

The number of drugs available for treatment of disease during the eighteenth century was very large. Fortunately, in the present context it is unnecessary to assess the pharmacological properties of these remedies, and one need only enquire whether there were improvements in therapy, either by introduction of new drugs or from more efficient use of existing ones, which are likely to have led to a reduction of mortality.

According to Singer, the only important drugs introduced between Hippocratic times and the beginning of the nineteenth century were laudanum, liver extract, mercury, cinchona, ipecacuanha and digitalis.[5] Mercury and cinchona were discussed in chapter 5 in relation to the infections, and laudanum, liver extract (in the circumstances in which it was then used) and ipecacuanha cannot be regarded as life-saving remedies. I must now consider the use of digitalis.

Even today digitalis adds only a few years to the life expectation of well chosen patients. The drug was included in the London Pharmacopeia of 1650, but was certainly used incorrectly before 1785, when Withering published his *Account of the Foxglove*, and can have had

[3] J. E. Ericksen, *On Hospitalism and the Causes of Death after Operations*. (London, 1874.)

[4] C. Singer, *A Short History of Medicine*. (Oxford, 1928), p. 162.

[5] C. Singer, 'Eighteenth-century medical science'. *British Medical Journal*, **1** (1951), p. 569.

little value before the nineteenth century, when Bright distinguished between dropsy of cardiac and renal origin. It is unlikely that digitalis made any substantial contribution to treatment of heart disease during the eighteenth century, and still more that it had any effect on mortality trends.

Among the drugs used in ancient medicine were many which are to be found in modern pharmacopeias. A few of these older remedies were of some value, but perhaps the only one which might now be regarded as potentially life-saving is iron. It was not valued greatly by Greek and Arab physicians, but was used widely in the seventeenth and eighteenth centuries. Sydenham and other physicians employed it as a tonic, and gave it in a variety of conditions which appear to have included some iron deficiency anaemias. It is impossible to express a confident opinion about what this treatment achieved, but it could have had no appreciable influence on the national death rate.

Hospitals and dispensaries

Great significance has been attached to the rapid growth of hospitals during the eighteenth entury. In 1700 there were two hospitals in London (St Bartholomew's and St Thomas's), and only five in the whole of England; by 1800 there were at least 50 hospitals in England, and according to Griffith accommodation available in London was nothing to be ashamed of, even when judged by modern standards.[6] But in assessing the contribution of hospitals to reduction of mortality we are concerned less with the number of beds than with the results of treatment of the patients who occupied them.

Griffith assumed that the growth of hospital accommodation was largely responsible for the steady drop in the death rate during the late nineteenth and early twentieth centuries, and concluded that hospitals must also have contributed materially to reduction of mortality in the eighteenth century. On present evidence it seems clear that neither the assumption nor the conclusion based on it is correct. The decline of the death rate during the nineteenth and twentieth centuries was not due mainly to medical measures. Perhaps the most useful contribution made by hospitals to the trend of mortality before 1900 was the isolation of infectious patients, first in separate wards of general hospitals and later in fever hospitals (mainly after the passage of the 1875 Public Health Act). But during the eighteenth and early nineteenth centuries, the importance of segregating infectious patients was not appreciated; it was believed that infectious and non-infectious cases

[6] G. T. Griffith, *Population Problems of the Age of Malthus*. Second edition, Frank Cass (London, 1967).

could be mixed in the ratio of one to six, and in 1854 persons infected with cholera were admitted to the general wards of St Bartholomew's Hospital.

Indeed, McKeown and Brown concluded that on balance the effects of hospital work in this period were probably harmful.[7] Contemporary accounts of the unsatisfactory conditions in eighteenth-century hospitals are available in the writings of Percival, Howard and others. The common cause of death was infectious disease; any patient admitted to hospital faced the risk of contracting a lethal infection. This risk existed until the second half of the nineteenth century, when Florence Nightingale found civil hospitals 'just as bad or worse' than military hospitals, and introduced her *Notes on Hospitals* with the well known observation, that the first requirement in a hospital is 'that it should do the sick no harm'. This objective was certainly not realized during the eighteenth century and it was not until much later that hospital patients could be reasonably certain of dying from the diseases with which they were admitted.

In the opening chapter I referred to criticism that this conclusion was inconsistent with data extracted from the records of an eighteenth century hospital, a suggestion which takes no account of the experience of hospitals in the present day.[8] Moreover, as Flinn has recognized, in the present context it is unnecessary to show that eighteenth-century hospitals increased mortality; it is sufficient if it is agreed that they did not reduce it.[9]

It is somewhat more difficult to assess the influence of the dispensary movement in the second half of the eighteenth century. The first London dispensary was founded in 1769, and 16 more were added before 1800. Unquestionably they brought treatment within the reach of a greater number of poor people, but whether the treatment was of any value is another matter. Few of the medicines available in the eighteenth century would now be judged to be effective; moreover, their usefulness was restricted by inability to identify the conditions in which they should be given and by lack of knowledge of methods of administration. The therapy administered from dispensaries was no better, even if no worse, than that provided in hospitals and private practice.

Yet it is possible that dispensaries made a more important, if less specific, contribution to health. According to Lettsom, they had a substantial effect upon sanitary standards, by teaching the importance of

[7] T. McKeown and R. G. Brown, 'Medical evidence related to English population changes in the eighteenth century'. *Population Studies*, **9** (1955), p. 119.

[8] E. Sigsworth, 'A provincial hospital in the eighteenth and early nineteenth centuries'. *Yorkshire Faculty Journal, College of General Practitioners* (June, 1966), p. 24.

[9] M. W. Flinn, *British Population Growth, 1700–1850*. Macmillan (London, 1970), p. 43.

cleanliness and ventilation.[10] Their contribution in this respect was comparable to that of obstetricians who advocated improvement in the hygiene of delivery.

To summarize: so far as can be judged from national statistics for England and Wales, all, or nearly all, of the reduction of mortality before the twentieth century was associated with a decrease of deaths from infectious diseases. However, national data do not include infanticide, which was probably an important cause of death until the last quarter of the nineteenth century. Various developments no doubt contributed to the decline of infanticide – foundling hospitals, a rising standard of living and maternal and child welfare services among others; but it seems clear that the most important influence was the use of contraception, from the late nineteenth century, to prevent the birth of unwanted children. Though probably less common, food deficiency diseases, including frank starvation, were other non-infective causes of death whose frequency decreased from the eighteenth century.

In the twentieth century, the contribution of non-infective conditions to the reduction of the death rate (they accounted for about a quarter of its decline) was also due to multiple influences. In several diseases therapeutic measures have been effective: for example, surgery in treatment of accidents and digestive illnesses, and obstetric and paediatric services in the care of the pregnant woman and newborn child. But a substantial part of the advance resulted from other influences, particularly improvement in nutrition of mothers and children. Without attempting to rank them in order of importance, I conclude that the main influences on the decline of mortality from non-infective conditions have been contraception, therapy and better nutrition.

[10] J. C. Lettsom, *On the Improvement of Medicine in London on the Basis of Public Good.* Second edition (London, 1775), p. 51.

9
Conclusions

Since the conclusions concerning the modern rise of population have been developed over several chapters, it will be desirable to bring them together in a general interpretation. I will begin by summarizing some of the main points made in the preceding pages.

1   When the rise of population from the eighteenth century to the present day is considered as a whole – and there are compelling reasons for this approach – it is seen to be a unique event which cannot be explained in the same terms as earlier population increases. Something happened which led to a greater and more prolonged expansion of population than any which preceded it (chapter 1).

2   The expansion was not due to an increase in the birth rate brought about by withdrawal of restraints on fertility. There is no evidence of this in developing countries today, or in developed countries since births and deaths were recorded reliably by national registration; indeed for most of the time birth rates have been falling. It is unlikely that there was a significant increase in fertility in the period preceding registration; but the issue is hardly of great importance to interpretation of the growth of population, since in Sweden its onset can have been no more than a few decades before births and deaths were registered (in 1749). Swedish data provide no evidence of a rising birth rate. The increase of population is therefore attributable to a decline of mortality (chapter 2).

3   The decline of mortality was due essentially to a reduction of deaths from infectious diseases. National statistics show this to be reason for the decline in England from registration (in 1838) until 1900, and it remains the predominant influence to the present day. It seems reasonable to conclude that the fall of mortality in the eighteenth and early nineteenth centuries was also associated with the infectious

diseases, although it is probable that there was a substantial decrease of deaths from two non-infective causes, infanticide and starvation (chapter 3).

4   While some infectious diseases may have declined as a result of a change in the character of the diseases brought about by modification of the relationship between organism and host, the enormous reduction of mortality and growth of population cannot be attributed to a fortuitous variation of this kind (chapter 4).

5   The fall of mortality was not influenced substantially by immunization or therapy before 1935 when sulphonamides became available. This conclusion is based both on knowledge of the role of medical measures in the present day, and consideration of the reasons for the decline of the major diseases which were associated with the reduction of mortality. The decrease of deaths from infections in which specific medical measures were effective earlier than 1935 – smallpox, syphilis, tetanus, diphtheria, diarrhoeal diseases and some surgical conditions – made only a small contribution to the total decline of the death rate after 1838 (chapter 5).

6   Exclusion of a fortuitous change in the character of infectious diseases and of immunization and therapy leaves one other explanation for the reduction of mortality, namely, improvements in the environment. The questions remain whether there are positive as well as negative grounds for this conclusion, and whether it is possible to specify the nature of the environmental influences.

7   From the second half of the nineteenth century a substantial reduction of mortality from intestinal infections followed the introduction of hygienic measures – purification of water, efficient sewage disposal and improved food hygiene, particularly in respect of milk. It is unlikely that such influences were effective before that time, since initially industrialization led to crowding and deterioration of hygienic conditions. However, the decline of infectious diseases which occurred progressively from the eighteenth century must have resulted in reduced contact with some infections as a secondary consequence of the diminished prevalence of the diseases (chapter 6).

8   The most acceptable explanation of the large reduction of mortality and growth of population which preceded advances in hygiene is an improvement in nutrition due to greater food supplies. The grounds for this conclusion are twofold. (a) There was undoubtedly a great increase in food production during the eighteenth and nineteenth

centuries, in England and Wales enough to support a population which trebled between 1700 and 1850 without significant food imports. (b) In the circumstances which existed prior to the agricultural and industrial revolutions, an improvement in food supplies was a necessary condition for a substantial and prolonged decline of mortality and expansion of population. The last point is in accord with present-day knowledge of the relation between malnutrition and infectious diseases (chapter 7).

9   The decline of mortality from non-infective causes of death (infanticide and starvation in the eighteenth and nineteenth centuries and a large number of conditions in the twentieth) was due partly to medical measures, but also to contraception and improvement in nutrition. Indeed, since the reduction of deaths from infanticide probably made the largest contribution to the decline, the change in reproductive behaviour which resulted in avoidance of unwanted pregnancies was probably the most important influence on the decrease of deaths from non-infective conditions (chapter 8).

Before attempting to bring these conclusions together in a general interpretation of the modern rise of population I shall consider briefly some of the related issues in the experience of other animals and of early man. Neither, it is true, has much direct bearing on interpretation of the growth of population in the past three centuries, when conditions of life were far removed from those in primitive societies and those for other animals in their natural habitats. Nevertheless, as a background to consideration of the modern problem it is useful, perhaps essential, to come to a conclusion concerning the determinants of health and population growth in the long period before they were modified by the changes which followed the first agricultural revolution. I refer to the relation between fertility and mortality, the common causes of death and experience of disease, particularly infectious disease.

The limited observations which have been made on animals in their natural habitats suggest that while reproductive rates and mortality rates have evolved by natural selection, they have not done so in balance, in the sense that numbers born are adjusted in relation to the capacity of the environment to support them. The objections to the alternative view – that fertility is restrained with regard for the resources of the environment, particularly its food supplies – have been outlined by Lack.[1] The most compelling objection to this interpretation is that it is based on the concept of 'group selection', the idea that by restriction of fertility animal populations maintain themselves around 'the level at which food resources are utilized to the fullest

[1] D. Lack, *Population Studies of Birds*. Clarendon Press (Oxford, 1966), p. 303.

extent possible without depletion'.[2] Since this implies that the majority of individuals born alive survive and reproduce, it is clearly in conflict with the Darwinian concept of natural selection. For 'group selection', if practised widely, would reduce or eliminate the ability of living things to adapt to a changing environment through natural selection, based on high and selective mortality.

The main causes of death among animals in their natural habitats are food shortage, disease and predation. According to Lack, 'the numbers of most birds, carnivorous mammals, certain rodents, large fish where not fished and a few insects are limited by food.' Numbers of some other animals, including gallinaceous birds, for most of the time are limited by predators, including insect parasites. But since predation results from the need for food, it is food supplies which directly through starvation or indirectly through predation determine the level of mortality and limit population size.

In view of the predominant part played by infectious diseases in the decline of human mortality during the past three centuries, it is important to note that disease is not a common cause of death in birds and other wild animals. Population sizes and densities of most animals are probably too low to maintain micro-organisms in the absence of an intermediate host. However, there are exceptions, particularly among arthropods, and it is significant that insects – the most numerous of the world's animal species – appear to have a central place in the history of viruses.

The level of fertility and causes of death of early man are of course unknown, and it is questionable whether the observations that have been made on the few peoples who have retained a primitive way of life to the present day have much bearing on the main issues. However, it is now possible to assess the feasibility of limitation of births in the absence of modern knowledge and techniques. Since a minimum weight for height is essential for the onset and maintenance of regular menstruation, it is likely that fertility was relatively low (as in some developing countries today) because of the prevalence of malnutrition. It is unlikely that early man was able to restrict fertility deliberately. In developing countries there is no evidence of control by the practice of continence; both experimental and epidemiological findings indicate that prolonged lactation is not a reliable means of avoiding pregnancy; and it is only in recent years in medical hands that abortion has become a safe and effective instrument. The method of undoubted effectiveness frequently discussed in this context is infanticide, but this is a postnatal rather than a prenatal influence.

[2] V. C. Wynne-Edwards, *Animal Dispersion in Relation to Social Behaviour*. Oliver and Boyd (Edinburgh, 1972), p. 132.

If restraints on fertility of early man were ineffective (except for the involuntary one imposed by deficient food supplies), it follows that the growth of the world's population was restricted by a high level of mortality. This conclusion is consistent with experience of developing countries today and of the advanced countries in the recent past. The common causes of death fall broadly into two classes, the first comprising those for which man is responsible (all forms of homicide, including war) and those for which he is not directly responsible, namely food deficiences, disease (particularly infectious disease) and injury arising from hunting and gathering. On the evidence available, or likely to become available, it is impossible to assess the relative contributions of these influences, which no doubt varied from one population to another and from time to time. What can be said is that all these causes are related to the environment, and particularly to its food supplies. For if homicide in its various forms was common, this was presumably determined ultimately by limitations of resources. And if starvation or infectious disease associated with food deficiency were important, they resulted even more directly from lack of food.

Viewed in this way, the common causes of death in early man were analogous to those outlined by Lack in his interpretation of the experience of other animals. In some, food shortage is the main 'mortality factor'; in others, food supplies set an ultimate limit to the growth of population, but the limit is not always reached because of other influences such as predation. With due regard for the deficient evidence and variable conditions, the experience of early man can be interpreted broadly in the same terms. At some times the level of mortality was probably determined mainly by shortage of food and associated disease; at other times the food limits may not have been reached because of a high death rate from causes such as infanticide and tribal war. This is consistent with the conclusion that the main restraint on population growth was a high level of mortality determined directly or indirectly by the availability of food.

There have been two major changes from the conditions of life of early man and both had profound effects on health and population growth. The first occurred about 10,000 years ago, with the domestication of plants and animals and the transition from a nomadic to a settled way of life; the second was associated with the agricultural and industrial developments of the past three centuries. Although we are concerned here mainly with the modern period, it is essential as a background to understand the effects of the changes associated with the first agricultural revolution.

The growth of early human populations was restricted by a high level of mortality determined by lack of food. The first agricultural revolution provided the food which made it possible for numbers to increase. Why then, presumably after an initial spurt, did the world's population rise so slowly that it was not until 1830 that it reached 1000 million? The answer to this question must be sought in man's experience of infectious disease at different periods of his history.

As already noted, disease, and particularly infectious disease, is not a common cause of death of animals in their normal habitats, probably because with few exceptions, they do not achieve the size and density of population required for the propagation and transmission of many micro-organisms. The same was broadly true of early man. He no doubt suffered from infections which are found in other primates, and from some contracted from animal vectors; but living in small groups he is unlikely to have experienced many of the diseases which are prominent today, particularly those which are airborne (such as measles, mumps, smallpox, tuberculosis, influenza, diphtheria and the common cold). The rise of airborne disease, including notably the respiratory infections, probably dates from the time when human populations first aggregated in groups of substantial size. This explains why infectious diseases became predominant as causes of death from the time of the first agricultural revolution.

To understand subsequent experience of the infections it is necessary to recognize that micro-organisms and man have evolved in balance, and that their relationship is changing constantly through the operation of natural selection in parasite and host. Hence, changes in the character of infectious diseases proceed continuously, and although related to the environment, are largely independent of recognizable influences such as medical measures, hygiene and nutrition. Moreover, the stability of the relationship is different for different organisms; for example it is very variable in the case of the streptococcus, less so in that of the tubercle bacillus or measles virus.

It is not to the advantage of a micro-organism to kill its host, and after a period of adaptation the two may settle to a relation of mutual tolerance, or, occasionally, advantage. However, disease or death may occur during the period of adaptation and, through natural selection, where the sickness of the hosts is a necessary condition for the dissemination of the parasites (as in the case of the coughs and sneezes which spread the cold virus or the diarrhoea which disseminates the cholera vibrio).

Another and critical influence is the state of nutrition of the host. Until recently it was not possible to establish unequivocably the relation between malnutrition and infectious disease, largely because populations which are undernourished are usually poor and suffer from multiple effects of poverty. It was particularly difficult to dissociate the effects of deficient food from those of increased exposure to infection. However, extensive experience in developing countries now leaves no doubt that malnourished populations have higher infection rates and are more likely to die when infected. Indeed, a recent report from the World Health Organization suggested that malnutrition was the most serious health problem among populations of developing countries, and that an improvement in nutrition was a necessary condition for a decline of infectious deaths and a general improvement in health.[3] Moreover, since we tend to think of malnutrition as manifested by the food-deficiency diseases, it should be emphasized that in developing countries it is not usually of the overt types such as rickets, beri-beri, pellagra and the protein-calorie deficiency syndromes, kwashiokor and marasmus; it is more often present as chronic malnutrition without specific features which are easily recognized.

In the light of these conclusions it is not difficult to interpret the reasons for the predominance of infectious diseases during the past 10,000 years. The increase in food supplies which resulted from the first agricultural revolution led to the growth of populations to the size and density needed for the propagation and transmission of micro-organisms. However, as the population continued to expand, food resources became again marginal, so that the relation between man and micro-organisms evolved over a period when man was, in general, poorly nourished. The relationship was unstable and finely balanced according to the physiological state of host and parasite; improvement in nutrition would tip the balance in favour of the former and deterioration in favour of the latter. In these circumstances an increase in food supplies became a necessary condition for a substantial reduction of mortality from infectious diseases, and limitation of numbers would have to follow if the reduction was to be made permanent.

These were the critical advances made in the western world in the eighteenth and nineteenth centuries. From about the end of the seventeenth century there was an enormous increase in food production, in Britain sufficient to feed a population which trebled between 1700 and 1850 with little supplement from imported foods. Although incidental to our theme, it is of great interest that this advance was due initially to the more effective application of traditional methods – increased land use, manuring, winter feeding, rotation of crops, etc. – rather than to mechanical and chemical measures associated with industrialization. Among the traditional methods, Hutchinson attached particular importance to the restoration of fertility through manuring,[4] and Langer assembled impressive evidence for the significance of the extensive cultivation of the potato and maize, introduced from the New World

[3] M. Behar, 'A deadly combination'. *World Health* (February–March, 1974), p. 29.
[4] Sir Joseph Hutchinson, 'Land and human populations'. *The Advancement of Science*, **23** (1966), p. 241.

in the seventeenth century.[5] Whatever the relative importance of the different advances there is no doubt that collectively they led to a great increase in food supplies which was later extended by mechanization, chemical fertilizers and, still later, insecticides.

Yet the improvement in health which resulted from the advances in agriculture would in time have been reversed, as that which presumably followed the first agricultural revolution was reversed, by increasing numbers, if the growth of population had not been restricted. But in France from the beginning of the nineteenth century, and in other countries somewhat later, the birth rate began to decline. In the same period food supplies continued to increase, and together the two influences maintained the favourable balance between food and numbers. Hence we owe the reduction of mortality and growth of population basically to improved nutrition which resulted from the increase in food and to the change in reproductive behaviour which ensured that the advance was not reversed.

The other major influence on the trend of the infections was reduction of exposure. As a primary influence, this was delayed until the second half of the nineteenth century, when men began to improve the quality of the environment. The initial advances were the purification of water, efficient disposal of sewage, and food hygiene, which together led to a rapid decline of intestinal diseases spread by water and food. Such measures had no effect on exposure to airborne infections, the diseases mainly associated with the reduction of mortality during the nineteenth century. However, in a period when infectious diseases are declining, for whatever reason, less frequent exposure follows as a secondary consequence of their reduced prevalence in the community. It is therefore probable that in the eighteenth and nineteenth centuries exposure to some infections decreased, as clearly it has in the case of tuberculosis in the twentieth century.

For the population as a whole this improvement secondary to lower prevalence must have been offset largely by deteriorating environmental conditions associated with industrialization; the crowding at home and at work in the industrial towns created ideal conditions for the spread of airborne diseases, and no doubt contributed substantially to the predominance of tuberculosis as a cause of death in the nineteenth century. But for the well-to-do, the advantages of reduced exposure as a secondary consequence of the lower prevalence of infectious diseases were not offset by deteriorating working and living conditions. This may explain, at least in part, the observation that life expectation of the aristocracy increased in the eighteenth and

[5] W. L. Langer, 'American foods and Europe's population growth, 1750–1850'. *Journal of Social History*, Winter Number (1975), p. 51.

nineteenth centuries, although they would be expected to offer little scope for the main influence on the general population, namely, an improvement in nutrition.

Finally, I must consider the part played by medical measures of immunization and therapy, long thought to be the main reason for population growth in the eighteenth century, and still considered significant by those attracted by the idea that inoculation led to a reduction of deaths from smallpox. In relation to the increase of population in the past three centuries the issue arises particularly in respect of the infections for, with the important exceptions of infanticide and starvation, until the twentieth century the decline of mortality was associated almost wholly with infectious diseases.

These are three lines of evidence which have led to the conclusion that medical measures had relatively little effect on the trend of mortality from the infections. First, there is increasing recognition that health is determined essentially by behavioural and environmental influences, and that the scope for effective medical intervention is limited. This is true not only of infections, but also of diseases such as cancer, chronic bronchitis and certain forms of heart disease, formerly thought to be intractable and now shown to be largely preventable by modification of behaviour and of the environment.

The second kind of evidence is derived from experience in developing countries, where it has been found that nutritional state is critical in determining the frequency and outcome of the infections. This is true even of diseases such as measles and whooping cough for which effective immunization is available, and indeed it is questionable whether infectious diseases can be controlled by immunization in a malnourished population.

The third line of enquiry has an even more direct bearing on assessment of the influence of immunization and therapy on the trend of mortality from infectious diseases in the period when they can be identified in national statistics, in Britain from the fourth decade of the nineteenth century. Examination of the diseases mainly associated with the fall of mortality shows that their death rates declined long before the introduction of effective immunization or treatment, and that by the time these measures became available the rates had fallen to a relatively low level. The diseases in which effective vaccination or therapy were available in the nineteenth or early twentieth centuries made only a small contribution to the reduction of mortality; it was not until 1935, with the introduction of sulphonamides and later, antibiotics, that medical measures became available which were sufficiently powerful to have an effect on national death rates. And even since 1935 they have not been the only or, probably, the main influences.

As mentioned earlier in this chapter, in Britain non-infective causes of death accounted for about a quarter of the fall of mortality in this century. But much the most prominent non-infective cause of death which declined was probably infanticide, which is believed to have been responsible for a high level of mortality in infancy until the late nineteenth century. The virtual disappearance of infanticide coincided with the reduction of the birth rate, and can be attributed credibly to the use of contraception to prevent unwanted pregnancies. Thus we owe this significant development to a change in behaviour, and consideration of other non-infective causes of death indicates that the main reasons for their decline were medical measures, contraception and improvement in nutrition. That is to say that the increase in food supplies and modification of behaviour were important influences on non-infective causes of death as well as on the infections.

Against this background it is possible to suggest an answer to the paradox which lies at the heart of interpretation of the rise of population: it is probable that the predominance of infectious diseases dates from the first agricultural revolution when men began to aggregate in populations of considerable size; why then did the infections decline from the time of the modern agricultural and industrial revolutions which led to the aggregation of still larger and more densely packed populations?

Population growth of early man was restricted by a high level of mortality due directly or indirectly to insufficient food. The increase in food supplies 10,000 years ago led to a reduction of mortality and expansion of population; the larger population created the conditions needed for the propagation and transmission of many micro-organisms, particularly those that are airborne. The population expanded to the level at which food resources became again marginal, so that the relation between infectious organisms and their human hosts evolved during a period when the hosts were, in general, poorly nourished. In these circumstances an improvement in nutrition was a necessary condition for a substantial and sustained decline of mortality and growth of population.

This condition was met in the eighteenth and nineteenth centuries. The great increase in food production from the end of the seventeenth century resulted in improvement in nutrition, and tipped the balance in favour of the hosts and against micro-organisms which cause disease. At this time however, and unlike experience 10,000 years earlier, numbers did not rise to the point at which food supplies again became marginal; food production continued to increase by the application of technology to agriculture; and even more important, population growth was limited by falling birth rates.

The greatly expanded populations of the industrial towns created ideal conditions for the spread of infectious diseases. The fact that mortality from the diseases declined in spite of these conditions indicates the critical influence of nutrition; a population which was fed better, if not adequately, was able to face the risks of increased exposure. Moreover, exposure to infection was limited in two ways: one indirect, as a result of the lower prevalence of the diseases; the other direct, following improvement in hygiene of water and food from the second half of the nineteenth century. The protection of milk was particularly important, for milk provides an excellent medium for the growth of micro-organisms and was largely responsible for the high level of infant mortality which continued until 1900.

There need be no disappointment with the conclusion that medical measures of immunization and treatment were relatively ineffective; they were also unnecessary. In the classical tradition there were two ideas concerning man's health: one, associated with the goddess Hygieia, that it could be achieved by a rational way of life; the other, personified by the god Asclepius, that it depended largely on the role of the physician as healer of the sick. Both concepts are to be found in Hippocratic writings, and they have survived in medical thought and practice down to the present day. However, since the seventeenth century at least, the Asclepian approach has been predominant. Philosophically, it derived support from Descartes' concept of the living organism as a machine which might be taken apart and reassembled if its structure and function were understood; practically, it seemed to find confirmation in the work of Kepler and Harvey and in the success of the physical sciences in manipulating inanimate matter. It is only in the past few decades that it has become evident that this interpretation is quite inaccurate, that the health of man is determined essentially by his behaviour, his food and the nature of the world around him, and is only marginally influenced by personal medical care. Intuitively we believe that *we are ill and are made well*; it is nearer the truth to say that *we are well and are made ill*.

In summary, there have been two major changes in man's way of life which had profound effects on his health and rate of population growth. Ten thousand years ago, the transition from a nomadic to a settled existence, with domestication of plants and animals, resulted in an increase in food supplies, a reduction of mortality and the growth of populations; but with unrestricted expansion of numbers food supplies again became marginal. The aggregation of large, malnourished populations created the conditions required for the propagation and transmission of micro-organisms, and so led to the predominance of infectious diseases as causes of sickness and death. This established a high level of mortality which limited the rate of population growth.

The chain of influences was broken during the eighteenth and nineteenth centuries when advances in agriculture brought an increase in food supplies. The improvement in nutrition which followed led to the decline of infectious diseases and to a reduction of mortality and growth of population. This advance, unlike the earlier one associated with the first agricultural revolution, was not reversed, because declining birth rates limited the growth of population and so maintained the favourable balance between food and numbers. An additional, and in a sense quite separate, influence was a reduction of exposure to infections, particularly intestinal infections, which resulted from improvements in the quality of water and food.

Index